A Caregiver's Guide for Dementia and Alzheimer's Disease

A Caregiver's Guide for Dementia and Alzheimer's Disease

A Caregiver's Guide for Dementia and Alzheimer's Disease

The Secret I Used to Love Someone With Cognitive Decline

Jenny Daniels

A Caregiver's Guide for Dementia and Alzheimer's Disease

© 2024 by Jenny Daniels
All rights reserved. No part of this publication may be reproduced, distributed, or transmitted in any form or by any means, including photocopying, recording, or other electronic or mechanical methods, without the prior written permission of the publisher. For information, contact:
jennycoy41@gmail.com

Disclaimer: This book offers general information on caregiving for dementia and Alzheimer's disease, based on the author's research and experience. It is not a substitute for professional medical, legal, or psychological advice. Readers should consult qualified professionals for guidance on specific health or legal issues related to caregiving.

While efforts were made to ensure the accuracy of information at publication, the author and publisher assume no responsibility for errors or for any consequences from using the information in this book.

Legal Notice: The author and publisher disclaim any liability for outcomes related to the use of this information. Readers should use their judgment and seek appropriate professional guidance.

References to specific products or treatments are not endorsements. This book does not establish a professional-client relationship between the author and reader.

A Caregiver's Guide for Dementia and Alzheimer's Disease

Gratitude

To My Amazing Readers,

Thank you for picking up this book! Caring for someone with dementia or Alzheimer's is no easy task; it's a rollercoaster of love, patience, and the occasional *"Where did I leave my own sanity?"* moment.

I wrote this guide to help lighten your load (and maybe make you chuckle when you need it most). You're doing incredible work, even on days it doesn't feel like it.

Take care of them, but don't forget to take care of you, too.

With love,
Jenny Daniels.

This book belongs to:

_____

_____

_____

A Caregiver's Guide for Dementia and Alzheimer's Disease

A Personal Note from Me to You

Caregiving is not just about tasks; it's about heart. I know this because I've been in your shoes. My late dad had dementia, and while it was one of the hardest journeys of my life, it was also one of the most meaningful. There were moments when I felt lost, overwhelmed, or like I wasn't doing enough but; there were also moments of deep connection, love, and even laughter.

As you read this book, I hope you find comfort in knowing that someone who truly understands wrote it for you. At the end, I've included some reflective questions to help you unpack your caregiving journey. (**Pages. 192-197**) Think of them as our way of having a conversation, one caregiver to another.

Take it one step at a time. You're doing better than you think.

With care,
Jenny Daniels.

Spread the Compassion

If this book touched your life, I'd love to hear your honest review, it helps others find it too.

Share it with friends, family, or anyone who might benefit. And don't miss my other books designed to inspire and uplift your journey.

Your support means everything. Thank you!

Caregivers are often the unsung heroes, quietly carrying the weight of responsibility and love.

Jenny Daniels

A Caregiver's Guide for Dementia and Alzheimer's Disease

FREE GIFT

Thank you for purchasing this book, I have lots free gift for you to help you navigate your journey as a caregiver, it helped me during my own journey too. You'll find it at the end of the book.

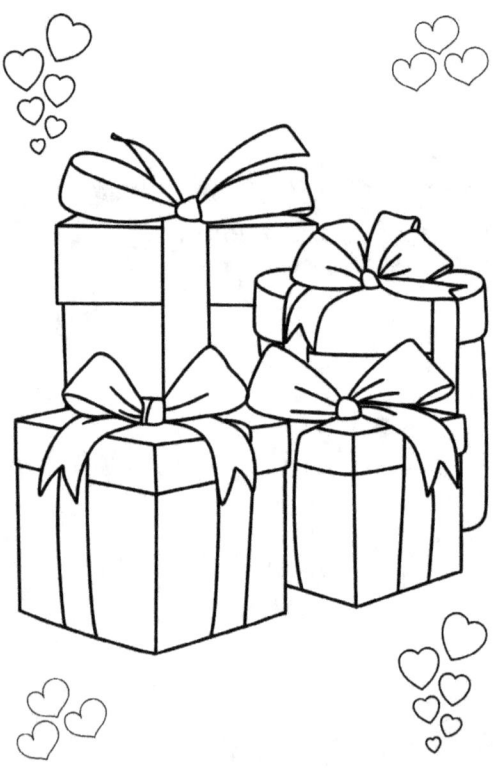

Dedication

To my dad, the only man who called me Margaret Thatcher because I fought so hard for him to still be alive but, all to no avail. (In loving memory.)

Table of Contents

How to Use This Book	13
Introduction	20
Why I Wrote This Book	21
The Journey	23
The Role of the Caregiver	23
Finding the Moments of Connection	24
Understanding Your Journey as a Caregiver	26
Setting Realistic Expectations	32
Early Stage	33
Moderate Stage	34
Severe Stage	35
Taking Care of Yourself	37
CHAPTER 1	**39**
Understanding Dementia and Alzheimer's Disease	39
Symptoms and Progression of Alzheimer's Disease	41
What Causes Alzheimer's Disease?	42
Differences Between Dementia and Alzheimer's Disease	43
Types of Dementia	44
Causes and Risk Factors for Dementia	47
CHAPTER 2	**50**
Recognizing the Early Signs and Stages of Dementia	50
Mild Cognitive Impairment (MCI):	52
Monitoring and Managing MCI	54
Stages of Dementia	54

The Importance of Early Detection	57
CHAPTER 3	**60**
Diagnosis and Assessment of Dementia	60
How Dementia is Diagnosed	60
Common Diagnostic Tests	63
Working with Specialists	64
What to Know About APOE-e4 and Other Genetic Markers	66
Planning After Diagnosis	67
CHAPTER 4	**71**
Building a Support System	71
Discussing the Diagnosis and Setting Boundaries	73
Involving the Person with Dementia	75
Finding Community Resources	76
Professional Support Options	78
CHAPTER 5	**81**
Daily Caregiving Essentials	81
Creating a Safe Living Environment	81
Establishing Daily Routines	83
Personal Hygiene and Dressing	85
Managing Medications	87
Food and Nutrition	88
Incontinence and Toileting Care	90
CHAPTER 6	**93**
Communication and Behavioral Management	93
Effective Communication Techniques	93
Understanding Behavioral Changes	95
Managing Sundowning and Sleep Disturbances	98

Coping with Hallucinations and Delusions 100
De-escalation Strategies 101

CHAPTER 7 — 104
Physical and Cognitive Health Management 104
Exercise and Mobility 104
Cognitive Stimulation Activities 106
Mental Health Care 108
Monitoring Health Conditions 109
Recognizing and Managing Pain 111

CHAPTER 8 — 113
Legal and Financial Planning 113
Legal Documents to Prepare 113
Financial Planning for Long-Term Care 115
Rights of the Person with Dementia 117
Making Decisions Together 118
Guardianship and Conservatorship 120

CHAPTER 9 — 124
Self-Care and Support for Caregivers 124
The Importance of Self-Care 125
Identifying Caregiver Burnout 126
Stress Management Techniques 128
Finding Time for Yourself 129
Counseling and Support Groups 131

CHAPTER 10 — 134
Advanced and End-of-Life Care 134
Transitioning to Full-Time Care 134
Hospice and Palliative Care 136
Emotional and Spiritual Support 138
Family Grief and Support 140
Legacy Planning and Bereavement 142

CHAPTER 11	**146**
Real-Life Stories and Case Studies	146
Lessons Learned from Other Caregivers	148
Finding Moments of Happiness in Caregiving	150
CHAPTER 12	**154**
Resources for Caregivers	154
List of Trusted Books on Dementia Care	154
Websites and Organizations	156
Apps and Tools	158
Templates and Checklists	160
CHAPTER 13	**163**
FAQs and Common Concerns	163
Answers to Frequently Asked Questions	163
Handling Caregiver Concerns	166
Conclusion	**170**
GLOSSARY	**175**
FREE GIFT	**181**
Emergency Contact Sheet	182
Medication and Healthcare Tracking Templates	184
Symptoms Tracker	186
Medication Tracker	188
Caregiver's Checklist	190
CONVERSATIONAL QUESTIONS	**192**
About The Author	**198**
INDEX	**200**

How to Use This Book

Navigating Chapters Based on Your Needs
Caring for someone with dementia or Alzheimer's disease is a deeply personal journey, and no two caregiving experiences look exactly alike. You may be facing a new diagnosis, navigating daily challenges, or preparing for the later stages. This book is meant to be a companion through all of these stages, designed to meet you where you are right now.

Whether you're reading from cover to cover or just skimming to find the right advice for the moment, this section will show you how to navigate each chapter. Use this guide to prioritize the sections most relevant to your caregiving situation. Feel free to skip around; this book is meant to be flexible, just like caregiving itself.

For New Caregivers
If you're just beginning the caregiving journey, you may feel overwhelmed by information, emotions, and the fear of what's ahead. These feelings are natural, and you're not alone. Start with Chapters 2 and 3.

<u>Understanding Dementia and Alzheimer's Disease:</u> This chapter will give you the foundational knowledge you need to understand the condition. By learning the differences between dementia and Alzheimer's and exploring the various types, you'll build a base for everything that follows. Think of this as laying the groundwork to make informed choices for your loved one.

<u>Chapter 2, Recognizing the Early Signs and Stages of Dementia:</u> When my dad first started showing signs of dementia, I remember how often I questioned myself: *"Is this just normal aging? Or is it something more?"* This chapter will help you differentiate between ordinary forgetfulness and early warning signs of dementia. You'll learn how to monitor symptoms, spot subtle changes, and take the first steps in getting a diagnosis.

After these chapters, you may wish to move into <u>Chapter 3, Diagnosis and Assessment,</u> which explains what to expect from medical appointments and cognitive tests. This will help you feel more prepared and confident as you advocate for your loved one.

For Caregivers Managing Daily Needs

A Caregiver's Guide for Dementia and Alzheimer's Disease

Once you're familiar with dementia and have received a diagnosis, you'll find yourself focusing more on day-to-day caregiving. Chapters 4 and 5 will be invaluable resources.

<u>Chapter 4. Building a Support System:</u> Caregiving is rarely a one-person job. This chapter walks you through creating a support system, from family and friends to local resources and professionals. After my dad's diagnosis, I thought I could handle everything alone. But as time went on, I realized the importance of asking for help. Building a care team will provide you with essential relief, helping you avoid burnout and focus on quality care.

<u>Chapter 5. Daily Caregiving Essentials:</u> Here, you'll find practical advice for structuring your loved one's day and creating a safe, comfortable environment. This chapter covers everything from medication management to personal hygiene. When you're in the thick of daily care, small tips; like using a pill organizer or finding soft clothing that's easy to put on, can make all the difference.

For Caregivers Dealing with Behavioral Challenges

As dementia progresses, you'll likely encounter behaviors that are confusing or even alarming, such as aggression, wandering, or repeated questions. These challenges require both knowledge and patience. Chapters 6 and 7 address these issues directly.

<u>Chapter 6, Communication and Behavioral Management:</u> Learning to communicate with someone who has dementia takes practice. In this chapter, you'll find ways to reduce frustration, use body language, and remain calm in tense moments. When my dad would get agitated, I learned that even a change in my tone or how I stood could make a difference. This chapter includes strategies for responding to behaviors that might otherwise escalate.

<u>Chapter 7, Physical and Cognitive Health Management:</u> It's not only the mind but also the body that dementia affects. This chapter offers advice on physical health, with ideas for gentle exercise and ways to incorporate stimulating activities, like puzzles or simple art projects. It also discusses recognizing pain and monitoring other health conditions. Simple adjustments, like creating a comfortable

seating area or introducing short walks, can significantly improve well-being.

For Long-Term Planning and Advanced Care
Planning for the future is one of the hardest parts of caregiving, but it's also necessary. These chapters will help you make important decisions and ensure your loved one is safe, comfortable, and honored in every stage.

Chapter 8, Legal and Financial Planning: The sooner you can address legal and financial planning, the better. Here, you'll find a breakdown of essential documents, from power of attorney to healthcare proxies, and advice on budgeting for long-term care. These details may feel overwhelming, but taking them step by step will protect both you and your loved one's interests.

Chapter 10, Advanced and End-of-Life Care: As dementia progresses into its later stages, care needs intensify. This chapter guides you through preparing for full-time care, whether at home or in a facility. Topics include hospice and palliative care options, emotional and spiritual support, and coping with grief. These sensitive issues are handled with compassion, giving you insight and options without judgment.

For Caregivers Seeking Emotional Support
Caregiving is physically and emotionally demanding, and it's normal to feel exhausted, overwhelmed, or even resentful at times. Chapter 9, Self-Care and Support for Caregivers, is specifically for you.

In this chapter, you'll find strategies to identify and manage caregiver burnout, including mindfulness practices, the importance of personal time, and ways to reach out for support. For years, I neglected my own health, thinking it was selfish to focus on myself. But I learned that taking care of myself made me a better caregiver. You'll also find advice on joining support groups, connecting with others, and finding moments of joy in the caregiving experience.

For Those Wanting Real-Life Insight and Practical Tools
If you're looking for real-life stories and tools to apply immediately, skip ahead to Chapters 11 and 12.

Chapter 11, Real-Life Stories and Case Studies: This chapter shares real accounts from other caregivers, capturing both the joys and challenges of caregiving. Reading about others' experiences can bring comfort and inspiration, reminding you that you're not alone in this journey.

Chapter 12, Resources for Caregivers: Here, you'll find books, websites, apps, and templates that can make caregiving easier. Whether you need a checklist for medication or an app to remind you of appointments, this chapter has practical resources you can rely on.

This book was written to offer you support, not to overwhelm you. Each chapter can be revisited as your needs evolve. Some days you may read in depth, while on others you might only have the energy to skim a few bullet points—and that's okay. This book will be here whenever you need it.

A Caregiver's Guide for Dementia and Alzheimer's Disease

Introduction

> ***What does it mean to watch someone you love slip slowly away into a world where you might no longer exist for them?***

If you're holding this book, you may already know that answer all too well. Dementia and Alzheimer's disease are not only hard on those who live with them but on those who care for them. My family and I faced this journey when my own father was diagnosed with dementia, and the experience left me profoundly changed. I know the worry, the endless questions, and the exhaustion that comes from caring for someone whose memories and abilities fade a little more each day. I also know the surprising moments of grace and connection that can still arise along the way.

When we first noticed my dad forgetting simple things, we brushed it off as "just aging." But as the memory gaps grew, so did my fear. Each new symptom felt like a door closing on the person I once knew so well. Like you, I found myself suddenly thrown into the role of a caregiver without a roadmap, trying to piece together how best to help someone I loved who no longer seemed to fully recognize me or our life together. Those were incredibly hard days, but they taught me valuable lessons that I hope to share with you in these pages.

Why I Wrote This Book

Caring for someone with dementia is unlike any other experience. It's often lonely, sometimes frightening, and always emotionally complex. I wish someone had told me at the beginning that it was okay to feel overwhelmed and that it was okay to grieve for the person who was slipping away, even if they were still physically with me. There were times I felt isolated, like no one could understand what I was going through. If that's how you're feeling right now, please know this: you are not alone. There is a vast community of caregivers who have walked this path, each struggling with the same mix of love, frustration, and exhaustion.

This book was written to help others like you navigate the difficult and often confusing journey of caregiving. It is here to offer practical advice, yes, but also to provide comfort and support. In the following chapters,

A Caregiver's Guide for Dementia and Alzheimer's Disease

I'll share the tools and strategies that made a difference for me, as well as insights from other caregivers who have walked similar paths. My hope is that you find in these pages both a guide and a companion.

The Journey

Dementia changes everything, but it does so slowly, piece by piece. Alzheimer's disease, the most common form of dementia, gradually affects memory, language, and behavior. Over time, you may notice changes in your loved one's personality and abilities. They may struggle with things that once came easily. But you'll also see that there are good days and bad days. This book will help you understand the progression of dementia so you can better anticipate these changes and prepare for the unexpected.

By understanding the journey from early symptoms to more advanced stages, you'll have a clearer picture of what lies ahead, as well as what your loved one is experiencing. I know that knowledge is only part of what you need, but it can help bring a sense of stability to an otherwise uncertain situation.

The Role of the Caregiver

As a caregiver, you take on a role that few people truly understand until they experience it firsthand. You become a protector, advocate, and companion to someone who may no longer be fully aware of what you're doing for them. It's a role that demands patience, resilience, and strength you may not know you have until you're tested.

But caregiving also has a way of bringing you face-to-face with your limits. Some days, no matter how hard you try, it may feel like nothing you do is enough. You might feel angry, frustrated, or even resentful; and then guilty for having those feelings. This is normal. If I've learned anything, it's that caregiving is a deeply human experience, with all the messiness, doubt, and courage that humanity entails. This book is here to remind you that you don't have to carry this burden alone and that there is no "perfect" way to be a caregiver. Each day, you're doing the best you can, and that is more than enough.

Finding the Moments of Connection

Throughout this journey, you may have days that feel more painful than others, but you may also discover moments of joy and deep connection that surprise you. There were times when my father would look at me with a familiar smile, as if they recognized me for just a brief second, and that moment would be enough to carry me through the next few difficult days. These little moments; whether it's a smile, a touch, or a flash of the person they once were, are gifts. They remind you of why you're here, why you keep going, and why your role as a caregiver matters so deeply.

As you read through this book, know that you are seen, your efforts are appreciated, and your courage is valued. Caregiving is one of the hardest things a person can do, but it is also one of the most meaningful. You may feel like you're losing your loved one, but in caring for them, you're showing them the most powerful love that exists: the love that endures through every hardship, every change, and every goodbye.

Let this book be your companion, your guide, and your reminder that you are not alone. Together, we'll walk this path with grace, patience, and hope.

A Caregiver's Guide for Dementia and Alzheimer's Disease

Understanding Your Journey as a Caregiver

When I first became a caregiver for my dad, I had no idea just how many layers of challenge I'd face. I knew it would be hard, but I couldn't imagine the daily strain, the exhaustion, and the constant weight of worry. Like most caregivers, I went into this journey because of love; deep, and strong love. But even love doesn't shield you from the toll that caregiving takes on every part of you.

If you're reading this, you may already be feeling it: the heavy, complex mix of emotions that hit you every day, the physical tiredness that clings to you, and the mental fatigue that doesn't seem to ease, no matter how much rest you get. This chapter is dedicated to helping you understand these challenges and recognize that you're not alone in facing them.

Caring for someone with dementia or Alzheimer's is a profoundly human experience, filled with both difficulties and unexpected beauty. And while there is no easy way through it, understanding the emotional, physical, and mental hurdles can give you the strength to keep moving forward.

Emotional Challenges: Grief, Guilt, and Love

One of the most heart-wrenching aspects of being a caregiver is that you're often grieving someone who is still physically present. As the dementia progresses, you may find yourself missing the person they used to be—the way they laughed, the stories they told, or the comforting feeling of their presence. But with each day, they may become a little harder to reach, and this sense of loss can feel endless. This kind of grief is complex because it doesn't have a clear end; it stretches across days, months, and years.

Alongside grief, you may also feel guilt. Perhaps you feel guilty when you lose your patience or when you wish for just one day to yourself. You may wonder if you're doing enough, if you're making the right decisions, or if there's something you could have done differently to prevent this disease from happening. I remember many nights lying awake, questioning myself, feeling guilty for the frustration I sometimes felt. But over time, I learned to accept that these feelings are natural. They don't mean that you love your person any less, they're just part of the human side of caregiving.

Still, despite the grief and guilt, there's an enduring, constant love that guides every action you take. It's this love that helps you find joy in the little moments—a smile, a laugh, or just the peace of knowing they're safe and cared for. The emotional journey of caregiving is like a patchwork quilt made up of every emotion you have, stitched together by love.

Physical Challenges: Fatigue, Health Risks, and Physical Care Tasks

Caring for someone with dementia is also physically demanding, often more so than people realize. There's the constant on-your-feet caregiving, especially as your loved one's mobility declines. You may be helping them out of bed, assisting with bathing, or even just staying vigilant, keeping an eye out to ensure they don't wander or hurt themselves. Each physical task, while a gesture of love, can be draining. It takes a toll on your body, especially if you're doing it day in and day out.

In my case, I found that the physical demands of caregiving were often underestimated. I didn't realize just how tiring it would be to keep up with daily routines, especially when my own energy levels were running low. And it's not just physical exhaustion; caregiving can impact your health. Studies show that caregivers are at greater risk of developing health issues themselves, including high blood pressure, weakened immune systems, and even conditions like heart disease. The stress can also lead to poor eating and sleep habits, especially when you're spending every ounce of your energy focused on someone else.

I learned the hard way that taking breaks and asking for help weren't luxuries, they were necessities. Your physical health is essential to your ability to care for your loved one, and I can't emphasize enough how important it is to prioritize your own well-being. It might feel selfish at first, but remember that you can't care for someone else if you're worn down and physically unwell. Give yourself permission to rest, to take walks, to nourish your own body. By caring for yourself, you are ultimately caring for your loved one, too.

Mental Challenges: Stress, Decision Fatigue, and Mental Overload
The mental strain of caregiving often comes as a surprise. There's an unrelenting stress that comes from balancing everything, managing appointments, keeping track of medications,

responding to behavioral changes, and constantly planning ahead for what might happen next. It's an endless to-do list that requires you to be alert, organized, and emotionally prepared at all times. Some days, it feels like there's no room left in your mind to even think, let alone rest.

This mental load also includes what many caregivers experience as "decision fatigue." The daily choices, big and small, can wear you down—decisions about their medical care, what foods to serve, or when to call in extra help. I remember how drained I felt from simply making all these choices, constantly worrying whether I was doing the right thing. There were days I doubted myself, wondering if I was missing something important or if I'd overlooked a better option. Decision fatigue is real, and it adds a level of mental exhaustion that often goes unacknowledged.

Caregiving for someone with dementia also involves enduring mental overload from the emotional shifts and uncertainties. One moment, your loved one may seem lucid and conversational, and the next, they might be confused, withdrawn, or even agitated. This unpredictability forces you to stay adaptable and alert, but it can also be mentally exhausting. You find yourself constantly adjusting, learning to expect the unexpected, and bracing yourself for whatever the day may bring.

If there's one thing I hope you take from this, it's to remember that your role as a caregiver, though heavy, is deeply meaningful. There will be days that stretch you to your limits and moments when you feel like you're carrying the weight of the world alone. But you are not alone. This journey is shared by millions of caregivers worldwide, each walking their own path yet connected by similar challenges and the same commitment to those they love.

Know that each day you care, each day you face these challenges, you're doing something extraordinary. You're giving someone who may not even recognize you the priceless gift of love and dignity. You're showing them that, even in the face of disease and loss, love endures. Take this journey one day at a time. You may not always feel it, but you are stronger than you know, and you're not walking this path alone.

Setting Realistic Expectations

If you're here, preparing to care for someone with dementia, it's crucial to understand that this journey will change both you and your loved one in profound ways. When my dad was first diagnosed, I was hopeful that we could manage things together, that maybe we'd find a rhythm that worked. But as the months and years passed, I came to realize how much dementia takes—slowly at first, and then more completely. Setting realistic expectations isn't about losing hope; it's about preparing your heart and mind for the unexpected, embracing the difficult days, and celebrating the precious moments that still appear along the way.

The Nature of Dementia's Progression
Dementia doesn't progress in a straight line. There were days with my dad that felt like gifts—moments where he'd recall a shared memory or look at me with clear recognition. Then there were times when he'd slip further away, losing pieces of himself, and I had to learn to let go of the version of him I'd known all my life. At every stage, I learned to adjust and adapt, recognizing that no two days would be the same. This journey requires flexibility, acceptance, and, above all, resilience.

A Caregiver's Guide for Dementia and Alzheimer's Disease

Early Stage

When my dad was in the early stages, the signs were easy to miss. He'd forget where he'd left his keys or call me by a different name, something I brushed off as just "getting older." But as time went on, I noticed more frequent lapses. Once, he forgot how to get to our favorite diner, a place we'd gone to every Saturday for years. That day, I could see the frustration and embarrassment on his face, and it was then I realized that he knew something was wrong too.

In these early days, I tried to support him without taking over. I'd remind him gently if he misplaced something, or I'd sit with him and go over stories from the past, hoping to ground him in memories that still felt familiar. It's a delicate dance at this stage, balancing their independence with the subtle support they need. I often reminded myself that he was still "him"—the same dad who raised me and loved me—and that my role now was to help him hold onto his dignity as long as possible.

Moderate Stage

As dementia progressed, it took a bigger toll. I remember one day in particular. He called me with panic in his voice, unable to remember which house he was in; even though he'd been living in that home for over a decade. When I arrived, I found him pacing the hallway, unsure of where he was supposed to be. He looked at me with a mix of relief and confusion, and in that moment, I felt the weight of our new reality: this wasn't something that was going to get better.

In the moderate stage, he needed more hands-on support, and I had to adjust my expectations quickly. He could no longer prepare meals safely, so I'd come by to cook for him, filling his fridge with easy-to-reheat dishes. I still miss his cooking and delicious meals. Honestly, my dad taught my mom most of the recipes she knows now. One evening, as we sat down to eat, he suddenly forgot how to use his fork. I watched him struggle, frustration building in his eyes, and my heart broke a little as I gently took his hand and guided it, helping him find his way again.

This stage was full of those small moments—when he'd forget my name or mistake me for someone else, when he'd lose his train of thought in the middle of a story, leaving both of us hanging in silence. I learned to listen without correcting him, to go along with his memories even if they were jumbled or incomplete. It wasn't always easy. There were days I'd leave his house feeling completely drained, unsure if I had the strength to keep up with all that he needed. But I discovered that what he needed most was for me to simply be there, to provide calm and reassurance even as everything else was slipping away.

Severe Stage

In the severe stage, everything changed. My dad could no longer recognize me or his surroundings, and he needed help with even the most basic tasks—eating, dressing, bathing. He'd often stare into space,lost in a world I couldn't reach, and sometimes he'd look at me with fear, as if I were a stranger. The most annoying part was when I prepared vegetable soup, which was his favorite and he told me that he doesn't eat it; my heart dropped.

Another time as I was helping him with breakfast, he looked up and asked, *"Where's my daughter?"* He didn't realize that I was right there beside him, the same person he'd taught to ride a bike, the same person who shared years of laughter and memories, the same little girl who he taught the Word of God through children's Bible videos. In that moment, I felt the full weight of loss—not just for him, but for both of us. And yet, I knew I couldn't dwell on that grief; he needed me to be fully present for him, so I put on a smile and reassured him, telling him I was right there.

This final stage was the most demanding. Every aspect of his care fell to me, and every interaction became bittersweet. He rarely spoke, and when he did, it was usually fragments of old memories, words that didn't connect but still somehow made sense to him. Once, while I was helping him get ready for bed, he looked at me and murmured, *"Thank you."* I don't know if he understood what he was thanking me for, but at that moment, those two simple words felt like the most meaningful thing I'd ever heard.

This stage taught me to let go of any expectations of improvement. It was about maintaining his dignity and comfort as best as I could, finding peace in the small gestures, like holding his hand or helping him settle in with his favorite old songs playing softly in the background. It was a time of constant goodbyes, but also a time of deep connection. I found a quiet strength in simply being there, providing the care he needed even when he couldn't recognize me.

Taking Care of Yourself

Through all these stages, I learned the importance of caring for myself, too. In the beginning, I tried to handle everything alone, but as his needs grew, I realized I couldn't do it all. I was worn down, both physically and emotionally, constantly fighting back tears or running on empty. Eventually, I found ways to balance his care with my own well-being. I joined a support group for caregivers, where I met others who understood the toll dementia takes on families. I leaned on friends and family, accepting help even when it was hard to ask.

Setting realistic expectations for yourself is just as important as setting them for your loved one. You will have days when you're patient and strong, and days when you're frustrated and overwhelmed. And that's okay. I learned to give myself grace, to let go of the guilt I felt when I needed a break, and to recognize that my own health mattered. Caring for my dad was a marathon, not a sprint, and I had to pace myself to see it through.

Dementia takes so much from both the person affected and their caregivers. But as hard as it was to see my dad lose his memory and his identity, I found peace in knowing that he was loved and cared for until the very end. This journey taught me a different kind of love—one that isn't defined by shared memories or words, but by presence, by the willingness to stand by someone even as they drift away.

Setting realistic expectations allowed me to accept each stage as it came, to adapt my care to his needs, and to find meaning in the small, often unnoticed moments. I learned that love doesn't depend on recognition or understanding; it's simply there, enduring through every loss and every goodbye.

As you step forward in your own caregiving journey, know that you, too, have this strength within you. There will be hard days, but there will also be moments that remind you of the bond you share and the love that remains.

CHAPTER 1

Understanding Dementia and Alzheimer's Disease

Dementia is a complex syndrome that impacts memory, thought, behavior, and the ability to perform everyday activities. It's not a specific disease, but rather a general term for a decline in cognitive function severe enough to interfere with daily life. One of the most well-known forms of dementia is Alzheimer's disease, but there are many other types. Understanding the differences among these types, as well as the risk factors and causes, can help us prepare for and adapt to the needs of those affected.

What is Dementia?
Dementia is a syndrome marked by a significant decline in mental abilities, affecting a person's ability to live independently. It's an umbrella term that covers various conditions, all of which involve the gradual breakdown of cognitive functions like memory, language, problem-solving, and reasoning. Dementia can range from mild to severe, and its symptoms typically worsen over time.

For a caregiver, this can be challenging and confusing because the decline doesn't happen overnight. I remember early on with my dad, there were little things—a forgotten name here, a misplaced object there—that didn't seem too concerning. But slowly, those small moments began to add up until it became clear that this was more than simple forgetfulness.

Dementia impacts nearly every part of a person's life. It's not only about memory loss but also changes in how they think, process information, and interact with others. When my dad began to lose the ability to follow conversations, I noticed he would retreat into silence, not out of disinterest, but because he was struggling to keep up. Understanding dementia means recognizing the invisible challenges the person faces every day.

What is Alzheimer's Disease?
It's a progressive disease, meaning that symptoms gradually worsen over time. Alzheimer's primarily affects memory, but as the disease advances, it impacts nearly all aspects of a person's functioning, including language, decision-making, and behavior.

Symptoms and Progression of Alzheimer's Disease

In the early stages, Alzheimer's disease is often marked by mild memory loss, especially of recent events. For instance, someone might forget conversations they had just a few hours earlier or struggle to recall where they placed a familiar object. They may also start losing track of time, forgetting dates, and struggling to plan or organize. In my father's case, he'd forget family dinners or show up at odd hours, thinking he was late.

As the disease progresses, memory loss becomes more severe, and other cognitive functions begin to deteriorate. Language difficulties emerge, making it hard to find words, follow conversations, or express thoughts. I remember one day my dad tried to tell me a story from his youth, something he'd done a hundred times before. But halfway through, he paused, lost in the memory he couldn't quite reach. It was like watching someone search for something precious in a fog, unable to find their way.

In the later stages of Alzheimer's, individuals may lose the ability to perform even basic daily tasks, such as dressing, eating, or recognizing loved ones. Eventually, they may lose the ability to speak entirely. My father's journey through these stages was a lesson in patience and adaptation, as we learned to communicate through touch and simple routines rather than words.

What Causes Alzheimer's Disease?

Alzheimer's disease is linked to abnormal deposits of proteins in the brain, which disrupt normal neuron communication and cause cell death. One protein, amyloid, forms plaques between neurons, while another protein, tau, forms tangles inside the neurons. The buildup of these proteins interferes with brain function, especially in areas involved in memory and planning. Over time, brain cells shrink and die, leading to the observable symptoms of Alzheimer's.

Genetics play a role in Alzheimer's, especially in rare early-onset cases that appear in people as young as their 30s or 40s. For late-onset Alzheimer's, which is more common, genetic factors, lifestyle choices, and environmental influences all contribute to the risk.

Differences Between Dementia and Alzheimer's Disease

It's important to understand that while all Alzheimer's disease cases are a type of dementia, not all dementia cases are Alzheimer's disease. Dementia is a broad term for cognitive decline, while Alzheimer's is a specific disease within that category. Think of dementia as an umbrella, under which Alzheimer's and several other types of dementia fall.

Alzheimer's disease and other types of dementia can differ in the symptoms and progression:

- **Onset and Symptoms**: Alzheimer's disease typically begins with memory loss, while other dementias might start with different symptoms. For example, Lewy Body Dementia often presents with visual hallucinations or movement issues before memory loss becomes apparent.

- **Progression**: Alzheimer's tends to progress in a more predictable pattern of memory loss, language decline, and loss of motor functions. In contrast, some forms of dementia may have fluctuating symptoms, or they may impact personality and judgment first, as seen in frontotemporal dementia.

- **Treatment Approaches**: While no cure exists for dementia or Alzheimer's, certain treatments may be more effective for some types than others. For instance, medications that target specific brain chemicals may alleviate symptoms in Alzheimer's, but they may not work as well for other forms of dementia.

Understanding these distinctions will help you set realistic expectations and prepare for the specific challenges that come with each type. In my father's case, knowing it was Alzheimer's gave us a clearer picture of what to expect, which, though difficult, helped us adapt.

Types of Dementia

Each type of dementia affects the brain differently, leading to distinct symptoms and progression patterns.

- **Alzheimer's Disease**: The most common type, affecting memory and gradually impacting all areas of life. Alzheimer's progresses through stages, from mild memory loss to severe cognitive and physical impairments.

- **Vascular Dementia**: This type is caused by reduced blood flow to the brain, often due to strokes or small blood vessel damage. People with vascular dementia may experience more sudden cognitive changes, such as trouble with organization, decision-making, or mood regulation. It's often accompanied by physical challenges, like difficulty walking.

- **Lewy Body Dementia**: Named for the abnormal protein deposits called Lewy bodies found in the brain, this form of dementia is unique because it often causes visual hallucinations, sleep disturbances, and movement issues similar to Parkinson's disease. Memory loss may be less pronounced initially, but fluctuating attention and alertness can be challenging for caregivers.

- **Frontotemporal Dementia**: Affecting the brain's frontal and temporal lobes, frontotemporal dementia often leads to dramatic personality and behavioral changes. People may become impulsive, socially inappropriate, or emotionally unresponsive. Language difficulties, such as trouble with speaking or understanding, are also common.

- **Mixed Dementia**: Some people have a combination of two or more types of dementia. For instance, someone may have both Alzheimer's and vascular dementia, leading to a blend of symptoms from both diseases. This can complicate treatment and make progression less predictable.

- **Rarer Forms (Creutzfeldt-Jakob Disease, Huntington's Disease):** While less common, some rarer forms of dementia also exist. Creutzfeldt-Jakob disease, caused by abnormal proteins called prions, leads to rapid cognitive decline and physical symptoms. Huntington's disease, a genetic disorder, also causes dementia, typically accompanied by motor impairments.

Causes and Risk Factors for Dementia

Dementia is linked to various risk factors, some of which are modifiable through lifestyle choices.

1. **Genetics**: Certain genes increase the risk of developing dementia, especially early-onset forms. For example, people with specific mutations in the APP, PSEN1, or PSEN2 genes have a high risk of early-onset Alzheimer's. In late-onset cases, having the APOE-e4 gene variant is associated with increased Alzheimer's risk, although it doesn't guarantee a diagnosis.

2. **Age**: This is the most significant risk factor for dementia, particularly Alzheimer's. While it's not a normal part of aging, the likelihood of developing dementia increases as people grow older.

3. **Heart Health**: The health of the cardiovascular system is closely linked to brain health. These health conditions such as high

blood pressure, high cholesterol, and diabetes can increase the risk of vascular dementia and Alzheimer's. Maintaining good heart health through diet, exercise, and stress management can reduce the risk.

4. **Lifestyle Choices**: Smoking, heavy alcohol consumption, lack of physical activity, and poor diet can all increase dementia risk. Engaging in regular physical exercise, eating a balanced diet rich in fruits, vegetables, and whole grains, and staying mentally and socially active can support brain health.

5. **Mental and Social Activity**: Keeping the mind active, whether through hobbies, learning new skills, or social interactions, may reduce the risk of dementia. While these activities aren't a cure-all, they can help build what scientists call "cognitive reserve," giving the brain more resilience against age-related decline.

6. **Environmental Factors**: Some research suggests that exposure to pollution, toxins, or head injuries may increase the risk of dementia. For example, people who have sustained multiple concussions may have a higher risk of dementia later in life.

Each type of dementia has its own path, its own set of challenges, and its own moments of heartbreak. For you, knowing what to expect and learning the underlying causes can provide a sense of direction amid the emotional chaos. For me, the more I learned about my father's condition, the better equipped I felt to handle each stage, even when it seemed impossible to bear.

CHAPTER 2

Recognizing the Early Signs and Stages of Dementia

Dementia develops gradually, and the symptoms may start subtly. Recognizing early signs and understanding how dementia progresses through its stages can help you plan and adjust your care. Early detection allows families to take action, make decisions, and seek interventions that may improve quality of life or slow the progression. In my experience with my father, noticing these early signs was a bittersweet revelation; it meant coming to terms with a new reality while holding on to the hope of making his life as fulfilling as possible.

Early Warning Signs: The early signs of dementia can be easy to dismiss as part of normal aging, especially since some symptoms are subtle at first. Here are some common early warning signs that dementia may be starting to develop:

1. Memory Issues: One of the earliest and most common signs of dementia is memory loss. However, this isn't just typical forgetfulness,

like misplacing keys or occasionally forgetting a name. People with early dementia may forget recent conversations, appointments, or important dates. For example, my dad would ask me the same questions repeatedly, not because he wasn't listening but because he genuinely didn't remember we'd already talked about it. He'd start getting frustrated, sensing something was wrong.

2. Language Problems: Struggling to find the right words or follow conversations can be another early sign of dementia. My father often paused in the middle of a sentence, as if searching through a fog for the words. This issue made him self-conscious and hesitant to speak up in family gatherings, leading him to withdraw.

3. Mood and Personality Changes: Dementia doesn't only affect memory; it also impacts mood and personality. People who are normally calm may become irritable or anxious. My dad, once easygoing, began to lose his patience more easily. Little things would frustrate him—like forgetting where he put his glasses or missing a detail in a story. These mood changes can strain family relationships, as it's sometimes hard to remember that these

outbursts are a symptom of the disease, not an intentional behavior.

4. Difficulty with Familiar Tasks: Another red flag is when someone begins to struggle with tasks they once managed easily. I recall my dad, who was always proud of his cooking skills, suddenly making mistakes in the kitchen. He'd add salt twice or forget a key ingredient in a family recipe he'd perfected over the years. At first, I thought he was just tired, but gradually, it became clear that his mind was struggling to follow the steps.

Mild Cognitive Impairment (MCI):

Mild Cognitive Impairment (MCI) is a condition that causes a slight but noticeable and measurable decline in cognitive abilities, including memory and thinking skills. While MCI doesn't always lead to dementia, it's considered a risk factor. Some people with MCI may stay at this stage for years, while others may eventually develop Alzheimer's or another type of dementia.

Symptoms of MCI

People with MCI experience cognitive changes that are noticeable but not severe enough to interfere with daily life. Symptoms may include:

- **Forgetfulness**: Similar to early dementia, but less severe. For example, forgetting details of conversations or appointments occasionally.

- **Trouble with Planning or Decision-Making:** Difficulty handling complex tasks or making quick decisions.

- Difficulty Following Conversations: Especially when there are multiple speakers or distractions.

For my father, MCI was the stage where we noticed he was becoming increasingly forgetful but could still handle most day-to-day activities. He might forget small details or need reminders, but he was mostly independent. It was only after several months that these symptoms became more pronounced, eventually leading to a dementia diagnosis.

Monitoring and Managing MCI

For those with MCI, close monitoring can help detect if cognitive abilities are declining further. Regular check-ups, memory exercises, and maintaining a healthy lifestyle can sometimes help delay the onset of dementia symptoms. We started keeping a family calendar and gently reminded my dad about upcoming events, which helped him feel supported without feeling like he was losing control.

Stages of Dementia

Dementia progresses through three primary stages: mild, moderate, and severe. Every stage presents a unique set of difficulties that call for changes to communication and caregiving techniques.

1. **Mild (Early Stage):** Initial Memory Lapses and Personality Changes

In the mild or early stage, people often experience memory lapses that go beyond ordinary forgetfulness. They might forget recent conversations, misplace items, or have trouble managing money or keeping track of bills. This is the stage when many people are first diagnosed.

This was the case of my dad too until we decided to establish a routine with him, setting up a daily schedule that helped him feel more in control and kept us aware of his needs.

2. **Moderate (Middle Stage):** <u>Increased Confusion, Behavioral Changes, and Need for Assistance</u>

As dementia progresses to the moderate stage, memory loss and confusion worsen. People may begin to struggle with familiar activities, have trouble recognizing familiar faces, and require help with tasks like dressing or bathing. Behavioral changes often become more prominent, including agitation, paranoia, or repetitive behaviors.

During this stage, my father's confusion deepened. There were days he'd forget where he was, and he'd panic, thinking he was in an unfamiliar place. He also became more withdrawn, preferring solitude over social interaction. At one point, he even became suspicious of my mother, thinking she was a stranger trying to take his things. This was one of the hardest stages for our family, as we had to learn to be patient, to stay calm, and to remind him gently of who we were without making him feel ashamed.

My dad's need for assistance also increased. Tasks like dressing became a challenge because he'd forget the order of putting on clothes or mix up the buttons and zippers. We learned to help him slowly, step by step, making the process as comfortable and respectful as possible. Small, routine tasks, like helping him comb his hair or guiding him to the kitchen for breakfast, became ways to show him he was loved because, he was loved.

3. **Severe (Late Stage):** Full-Time Care, Physical Decline, and Non-Verbal Stages

In the severe stage, dementia impacts nearly every aspect of a person's functioning. People may lose the ability to walk, speak, or even eat independently. Full-time care is usually necessary at this stage, as the person may no longer recognize loved ones or respond to communication.

When my father reached this stage, he could no longer speak, but he would hold our hands with a grip that told us he knew we were there. Even though he couldn't recognize me as his daughter, I knew that he sensed our presence. We communicated through gentle touches, shared silences, and familiar music. He would respond to some songs from his younger days with a soft smile, a reminder that somewhere inside, he still remembered.

As his physical health declined, we had to assist him with every daily task, from feeding to moving him in bed to prevent bedsores. It was emotionally and physically demanding, but caring for him at that stage became an act of devotion. The person he once was might have faded, but he was still our family, and he deserved love and dignity to the very end.

The Importance of Early Detection

Detecting dementia in its early stages is crucial, as it offers several benefits for both the individual and the family.

1. **Access to Treatment and Support:** Early diagnosis allows for early intervention, including medications that may help manage symptoms temporarily. Although there's no

cure for dementia, certain drugs can slow down the progression, particularly in Alzheimer's disease. Early intervention also connects families with support resources, such as counseling, educational programs, and support groups, which can be vital in preparing for what lies ahead.

2. **Planning for the Future**: When dementia is diagnosed early, the person affected can participate in planning for their future care. This includes legal decisions, such as setting up a power of attorney or health care proxy, and financial planning. It was important for our family to have my dad's input on these matters before his condition worsened. He shared his wishes for end-of-life care and ensured that his finances were in order. Having those conversations early on was emotionally difficult, but they became a source of comfort later, knowing we were honoring his wishes.

3. **Emotional Preparation and Relationship Building:** Early detection provides time for family members to emotionally prepare and make the most of the time they have together. In those early years, we focused on spending quality time with my father. We'd look through old photo albums,

reliving memories and sharing stories. This time allowed us to create a legacy of love and connection that carried us through the harder days.

4. **Adapting Daily Routines and Environments:** With early diagnosis, families can begin making practical changes to the home to improve safety and accessibility. For instance, we removed tripping hazards, added nightlights to prevent falls, and installed handrails in the bathroom. These small changes helped us ensure that Dad could live safely at home as long as possible.

Recognizing the early signs and understanding the stages of dementia will give you the insight and tools you need to offer compassionate and adaptive care.

The lessons I learned caring for my father taught me not only about dementia but about patience, acceptance, and the power of human connection.

CHAPTER 3

Diagnosis and Assessment of Dementia

Receiving a dementia diagnosis is often a long, emotional process involving multiple tests, specialists, and discussions with family. Early and accurate diagnosis is essential for planning, accessing support, and understanding what lies ahead. My father's journey to a diagnosis was both confusing and emotional for all of us; it involved learning a lot about medical procedures and tests we had never heard of before. Here, we'll break down the key components of dementia diagnosis, from the initial assessments to working with specialists, and explore what families can expect once a diagnosis is confirmed.

How Dementia is Diagnosed

Cognitive Tests, MRI, PET Scans, and Medical History

Diagnosing dementia isn't straightforward. There's no single test for dementia, so doctors use a combination of assessments to determine the cause and progression of symptoms. My dad's journey began with a few noticeable memory lapses, but it wasn't until he became confused in familiar places that we realized we needed medical advice. The diagnosis process includes the following steps:

1. **Cognitive Tests:** Cognitive tests evaluate a person's memory, problem-solving skills, language, and thinking abilities. These tests are usually one of the first steps in diagnosing dementia, and they're designed to measure changes in thinking patterns and memory retention. I remember watching my dad try to recall a list of words the doctor had given him just a few minutes earlier, and the frustration he felt when he couldn't. Cognitive tests were one of the earliest clues that he might be dealing with something beyond normal aging.

2. **Brain Imaging (MRI and PET Scans):** MRI (Magnetic Resonance Imaging) and PET (Positron Emission Tomography) scans provide a closer look at the brain's structure and function. MRI scans can reveal shrinkage in certain brain areas, while PET scans show how glucose is used in the brain, indicating areas with decreased activity. In Dad's case, the doctor suggested an MRI after his cognitive tests showed notable decline. The results

showed shrinkage in areas associated with memory, which supported the diagnosis of dementia.

3. **Medical History and Family Interviews:** Gathering information about the patient's medical history and family observations is crucial. The doctor asked us detailed questions about my dad's health, past illnesses, and any family history of dementia. Having the family involved helped fill in gaps, as Dad couldn't always remember the details himself. Describing our observations helped the doctor understand his symptoms better and gave insight into how he was coping daily.

4. **Blood Tests and Physical Exams**: Sometimes, certain physical conditions—like vitamin deficiencies, thyroid problems, or infections—can mimic dementia symptoms. Blood tests help rule out these other causes. Although this wasn't the case for my father, it's reassuring to know that these steps are taken to ensure nothing is overlooked.

Each part of this process felt like a step closer to understanding what my dad was facing. The combination of tests helped build a clearer picture, allowing us to prepare for the journey ahead.

Common Diagnostic Tests

Two of the most commonly used cognitive tests in diagnosing dementia are the Mini-Mental State Exam (MMSE) and the Montreal Cognitive Assessment (MoCA). Both tests assess memory, attention, language, and orientation, but they serve different purposes and can highlight various aspects of cognitive decline.

1. Mini-Mental State Exam (MMSE): The MMSE is a brief, widely used test that scores cognitive function on a scale from 0 to 30. It includes tasks like recalling a list of words, identifying objects, and performing basic math problems. My father's doctor used this test as one of the first assessments. Watching Dad struggle with some of the questions was painful, but it gave us a concrete sense of how much he was already struggling with memory and recall. The MMSE doesn't diagnose dementia on its own, but it helps indicate how far cognitive decline may have progressed.

2. <u>Montreal Cognitive Assessment (MoCA)</u>: The MoCA is similar to the MMSE but includes additional tasks to detect mild cognitive impairment (MCI) more accurately. It includes activities such as drawing a clock, naming animals, and listing as many words as possible starting with a certain letter. My dad found parts of the MoCA challenging, especially the language tasks, but it highlighted the areas where he needed the most help. The MoCA helped identify early symptoms that might have been missed with other tests.

These tests are valuable tools for both families and doctors, offering a benchmark for tracking changes in cognitive abilities over time.

Working with Specialists

Diagnosing and managing dementia often involves a team of specialists, each bringing unique expertise. Our family quickly learned that treating dementia wasn't a one-person job. Here are the key specialists typically involved:

1. **Geriatricians**: Geriatricians are doctors who specialize in the health issues of older adults. They understand the complexities of aging and the unique needs of dementia

patients. My dad's geriatrician was the first to notice patterns in his symptoms and recommended further tests. Geriatricians often guide families on managing the general health needs of a dementia patient, like nutrition, physical activity, and medications.

2. **Neurologists**: Neurologists specialize in disorders of the brain and nervous system. They play a critical role in diagnosing the type of dementia a patient may have. My father's neurologist helped us understand the physical changes happening in his brain. The neurologist also ordered MRI and PET scans, which confirmed that parts of my dad's brain were shrinking. This confirmation gave us clarity, as we could finally understand why he was struggling with memory and tasks he'd done all his life.

3. **Psychologists** and Psychiatrists: Psychologists and psychiatrists help address the behavioral and emotional aspects of dementia. My father went through a phase of agitation and paranoia, and working with a psychologist helped us learn ways to respond and de-escalate situations. They can also provide support to family members dealing with the stress and emotional toll of caregiving.

Working with this team gave us a sense of partnership. These specialists guided us through difficult decisions and helped us understand what was happening, step by step.

What to Know About APOE-e4 and Other Genetic Markers

Genetic testing can offer some insight into dementia risk, particularly for Alzheimer's disease. Although not every case of dementia is hereditary, certain genetic markers are associated with a higher likelihood of developing Alzheimer's.

1. APOE-e4 Gene: One of the most well-known genetic markers is the APOE-e4 gene. People who inherit one or two copies of this gene variant have a higher risk of developing Alzheimer's, although it's not a guarantee. Having the APOE-e4 gene doesn't mean someone will definitely get dementia, but it can increase susceptibility. We discussed genetic testing with my dad's doctor, but ultimately decided against it, as it wouldn't change the course of treatment.

2. Other Genetic Markers: In rare cases of early-onset Alzheimer's, specific mutations in

the APP, PSEN1, and PSEN2 genes can directly cause the disease. These cases tend to occur in people younger than 65. Our family was fortunate that Dad's condition wasn't caused by these genes, but for families with a history of early-onset dementia, genetic counseling and testing can be useful in planning and understanding the risk for future generations.

3. Biomarkers: In addition to genetic markers, certain biomarkers in the blood, spinal fluid, or brain imaging can indicate the presence of dementia. For example, higher levels of amyloid and tau proteins in cerebrospinal fluid are linked to Alzheimer's. Biomarkers can be useful in confirming a diagnosis, especially in research settings, but they're not widely available as routine tests.

Although genetic testing and biomarkers are still developing fields, they hold promise for improving early diagnosis and personalized treatments in the future.

Planning After Diagnosis

A dementia diagnosis marks the beginning of a new journey, and families often wonder what to do next. Planning after diagnosis involves practical steps, emotional preparation, and setting realistic expectations for the future.

- **Discuss Care Options Early**: After my father's diagnosis, one of the first things we did was sit down as a family to discuss care options. Would he stay at home? Would he eventually need residential care? These conversations were tough, but having his input helped us understand his wishes. Early discussions allow the person with dementia to share their preferences while they're still able to participate.

- **Legal and Financial Planning:** Dementia gradually affects a person's decision-making abilities, so it's crucial to organize legal and financial matters early. This might include setting up a power of attorney, healthcare proxy, or creating an advance directive. My father, for example, wanted to ensure his finances were in order, so we worked together to manage his accounts and establish a power of attorney. This way, he could have peace of mind, and we could ensure his wishes were honored.

- ***Establish a Support System***: Dementia caregiving is demanding, and no one should do it alone. We found that building a support system was essential. Family members, friends, local organizations, and healthcare professionals all became part of our care network. We also connected with local support groups, which allowed us to share experiences with other families going through similar situations.

- ***Prepare Emotionally and Set Expectations:*** Receiving a dementia diagnosis can be overwhelming, but it also gives families time to adjust and prepare. Setting realistic expectations is key. We knew that my dad's condition would gradually worsen, and while this was difficult to accept, it helped us be more patient. This is also a time to focus on creating meaningful moments, whether it's going through old photo albums, cooking favorite recipes, or simply enjoying time together. These small memories became cherished reminders of the bond we shared.

- ***Plan for the Future Stages of Care***: As dementia progresses, care needs increase. Planning for each stage—whether it's modifying the home environment, hiring additional support, or transitioning to full-time care—can ease the process. We started by making small adjustments at home, like labeling drawers and placing familiar objects in easy-to-find locations. Eventually, we discussed options for long-term care, knowing it might become necessary later on.

A dementia diagnosis is never easy, but understanding the diagnosis and assessment process, working with specialists, and planning ahead can help families cope with the journey.

CHAPTER 4

Building a Support System

Dementia caregiving can be overwhelming, especially as the needs of a person with dementia grow over time. One of the most important things for you as a caregiver to do is to build a strong support system, a network of people and resources that can provide help, guidance, and emotional support. For our family, creating this support system around my dad was essential. It allowed us to share responsibilities, reduce burnout, and maintain a sense of normalcy in our lives.

Creating a Care Team
A care team is a group of people who come together to share caregiving responsibilities. This team often includes family members, friends, healthcare professionals, and sometimes, outside help such as respite care providers. Building a care team early on can ease the caregiving burden and ensure that there's always someone available to help.

1. Family and Friends: Family members are often the first people to join a care team. In our family, we divided tasks to avoid overwhelming

any one person. I took on coordinating appointments and medications, while my siblings helped with meal prep and household tasks. Friends also offered support in smaller ways, sometimes they'd sit with my dad so we could get a break, or they'd help with errands. These small contributions were a lifeline.

2. Healthcare Professionals: The support of healthcare providers is crucial. This includes the person's primary doctor, specialists like neurologists, and sometimes physical therapists or psychologists. My dad's neurologist was part of our care team, guiding us through the progression of his dementia and adjusting his medications as needed. Having a regular point of contact with these professionals helped us navigate each stage of his illness with more confidence.

3. Respite Care: Respite care provides temporary relief for caregivers by allowing someone else to care for the person with dementia. For us, respite care came in the form of an adult day program where my dad could spend a few hours a week engaging in activities, socializing, and receiving supervised care. This time allowed us to rest, run errands, and simply take a mental break. Having these

moments of relief helped prevent burnout and gave us the energy to return to caregiving with renewed patience.

Creating a care team not only eased the workload but also provided emotional support. We felt that we weren't alone in the journey, and knowing there was always someone to rely on made a huge difference.

Discussing the Diagnosis and Setting Boundaries

Talking about a dementia diagnosis can be difficult, especially with family and friends who may not fully understand what the diagnosis means. However, clear communication is essential for creating a supportive environment and setting realistic expectations about what care will look like.

1. Discussing the Diagnosis: Sharing the diagnosis openly helps family and friends understand the challenges and prepare for the changes ahead. When we told my dad's siblings and friends, we were upfront about his condition and explained what he might need as his illness progressed. We emphasized that dementia isn't just memory loss but also

involves changes in mood, behavior, and physical abilities. This conversation opened the door for others to step in and help, as they understood what we were going through.

2. Setting Boundaries: As much as family and friends may want to help, it's essential to set boundaries. Caregiving can be exhausting, and not everyone is able or willing to provide the same level of support. I remember a close friend offering to visit weekly, but we agreed that we'd let her know if and when my dad was up for company. Setting boundaries allowed us to manage my dad's energy levels and gave him the space he needed, without offending those who wanted to help.

3. Creating a Communication Plan: With so many people involved, keeping everyone informed can be a challenge. We found it helpful to set up a group message or regular email updates to share information about my dad's condition, his appointments, and any specific needs. This way, family members stayed updated and knew when we needed help without us having to call each person individually.

Involving the Person with Dementia

As dementia progresses, a person's ability to make decisions may decline, but involving them in care decisions early on is both respectful and empowering. Including them in the process allows them to retain a sense of control and dignity.

1. Respecting Their Independence: In the early stages of my dad's illness, he was still able to express his preferences about his care. We sat down together and talked about his wishes for the future, including his desire to stay at home as long as possible and which family members he preferred to handle certain tasks. This conversation gave us clarity and provided him with the assurance that we respected his autonomy.

2. Adapting as Needs Change: As my dad's symptoms worsened, we adjusted our approach, involving him in simpler decisions like choosing his clothes or deciding on activities for the day. Although he couldn't make complex choices, these small decisions gave him a sense of normalcy. Maintaining his involvement in daily life reminded us that he

was still an active part of our family, not just someone who needed care.

3. Supporting Their Dignity: Involving the person with dementia in decisions is not just practical—it's a way to honor their dignity. Allowing my dad to express his preferences in small ways, even in the later stages, made him feel valued. He may have forgotten the conversations, but we believe that sense of respect and involvement gave him comfort.

Finding Community Resources

Connecting with local and online resources can provide caregivers with valuable support, education, and a sense of community. These resources were crucial for our family, providing us with information and emotional support through each stage of my dad's illness.

1. Local Support Groups: Support groups bring together people facing similar challenges, creating a space for sharing experiences and learning from others. Attending a support group was one of the most helpful things we did. Hearing from other caregivers who were dealing with similar situations provided us with

practical tips, and it was comforting to know we weren't alone.

2. Community Centers and Adult Day Programs: Many community centers offer adult day programs where people with dementia can engage in activities, exercise, and social interaction under supervision. My dad enjoyed these visits; he'd participate in group activities, and the change of scenery often lifted his spirits. Meanwhile, it gave us a break and reassurance that he was in a safe and stimulating environment.

3. Online Resources: Online support groups, forums, and websites are also valuable, especially for caregivers who may not have local resources nearby. We found online communities helpful for specific questions, like tips for managing behavioral changes or ideas for activities that could engage my dad. These resources provided immediate access to advice from people all over the world, many of whom had valuable insights to share.

4. Educational Workshops and Classes: Many organizations offer classes and workshops for caregivers, covering topics such as managing daily care, handling behavioral changes, and

understanding the progression of dementia. Attending these classes equipped us with practical tools and helped us feel more prepared.

Community resources offer both practical help and emotional support, making a difficult journey feel a bit more manageable. These connections became lifelines, reminding us that we were part of a larger network of caregivers facing similar struggles.

Professional Support Options

Professional support can provide caregivers with essential relief and expertise. For us, seeking professional help was an investment in both my dad's well-being and our family's peace of mind.

1. Home Health Aides: Home health aides assist with daily tasks such as bathing, dressing, and feeding. They're trained to support people with dementia, making them valuable members of the care team. We brought in a home health aide for a few hours a day, which gave us time to rest and tend to our own needs while knowing my dad was in capable hands. This support allowed us to

focus on our relationship with him instead of being consumed by caregiving duties.

2. Geriatric Care Managers: Geriatric care managers are professionals who help families navigate the complexities of elder care, including coordinating medical appointments, assessing home safety, and connecting families with resources. Our care manager helped us with organizing appointments, managing medications, and keeping track of my dad's overall health. She became a reliable resource for questions and provided us with practical solutions for his changing needs.

3. Therapy and Counseling: Caregiving can be emotionally exhausting, and therapy can provide caregivers with a safe space to process their feelings and manage stress. I attended counseling sessions myself to work through the emotional toll of seeing my dad's decline and learning to balance caregiving with my own life. These sessions helped me build resilience, gain perspective, and stay emotionally grounded, allowing me to be a more patient and effective caregiver.

4. Palliative Care Services: As dementia progresses, palliative care can provide

comfort-focused support for the person with dementia. These services focus on managing pain and improving quality of life. We began incorporating palliative care when my dad's physical condition declined, ensuring he was comfortable and as free of pain as possible.

Through each step, our family found strength, resilience, and a deepened sense of connection; reminders that even amid the challenges, love and support remain at the heart of this journey.

CHAPTER 5

Daily Caregiving Essentials

Caring for someone with dementia is a continuous process that evolves as the disease progresses. While the needs of your loved one may change, having a foundation of daily caregiving essentials can help provide structure, comfort, and dignity. Creating a safe, consistent, and supportive environment will make everyday tasks easier for both the caregiver and the person with dementia. Each of these caregiving essentials is based on my experiences with my dad and the valuable lessons our family learned while helping him navigate his journey.

Creating a Safe Living Environment

Safety in the home becomes increasingly important as dementia progresses. Dementia can cause confusion, poor judgment, and decreased motor skills, which increase the risk of accidents. For our family, adapting our home to minimize these risks was essential in creating a safe space for my dad.

- **Reducing Fall Risks**: Falls are one of the biggest safety concerns for people with dementia. To prevent falls, we removed rugs that could slip, cleared clutter, and ensured that furniture was arranged to create wide, open pathways. We also added grab bars in the bathroom and next to the bed, making it easier for my dad to steady himself. These small adjustments made him feel more comfortable moving around without fear.

- **Monitoring Hazards:** Dementia can lead people to forget important safety habits, such as turning off the stove or locking the doors. To prevent accidents, we placed covers on the stove knobs, used automatic shut-off devices, and labeled frequently used cabinets to reduce confusion. We also installed locks high on exterior doors since my dad sometimes wandered and might accidentally go outside unsupervised.

- **Using Assistive Devices**: Assistive devices can promote independence while ensuring safety. For example, we provided my dad with a walker that gave him support as he moved around the house. In order to gently notify us if he woke up throughout the night, we later installed a bed alarm. These devices became a part of our daily routine, giving my dad the mobility and dignity he valued while keeping us aware of his movements.

Creating a safe home environment allowed us to relax, knowing my dad could navigate his surroundings without fear of injury. Making these adjustments early made our home feel less like a maze of hazards and more like a space where he could live as independently as possible.

Establishing Daily Routines

For people with dementia, structure and familiarity are incredibly comforting. A consistent daily routine provides a sense of stability, reducing anxiety and confusion. We found that establishing predictable routines for my dad helped him feel secure and gave us a framework for managing each day.

1. Regular Meal Times: Setting regular meal times helped us create a rhythm for the day.

We found that eating at the same time each day gave my dad something to look forward to and helped him maintain his appetite. When he occasionally forgot he'd already eaten, we gently reminded him, focusing on familiar foods he enjoyed, like his favorite breakfast oatmeal. Serving meals in a quiet, distraction-free environment also helped him stay focused.

2. Bathing Routine: Bathing can be challenging for those with dementia, who may resist or fear it. Setting up a regular bathing schedule made it feel less like an unpredictable task. We chose mornings for his showers, keeping the bathroom warm and using calming, familiar scents. Talking through each step and using simple instructions, like "Let's rinse your arms now," helped reduce his anxiety and keep the process smooth.

3. Bedtime Routine: Consistent bedtime routines made a big difference in my dad's sleep quality. Each night, we followed a series of steps: lowering the lights, playing soft music, and sitting with him to read or talk quietly. This gentle transition into bedtime helped him settle more easily and reduced restlessness.

Once he got into a regular sleep pattern, his overall mood improved during the day.

Establishing these routines gave my dad a comforting structure, and it allowed us to anticipate his needs. We learned that having consistent daily practices helped him feel oriented and reduced the stress he felt when unfamiliar tasks popped up.

Personal Hygiene and Dressing

Maintaining personal hygiene and dressing is an essential part of daily life, but dementia can make these tasks challenging. Encouraging independence while providing support can help preserve a sense of dignity and self-confidence.

1. Step-by-Step Guidance: We learned that breaking tasks into simple steps made it easier for my dad to participate in his hygiene routine. Instead of overwhelming him with multiple tasks, we'd guide him through each step, one at a time. For example, we'd start with brushing his teeth, then move to washing his face, and finally help him comb his hair. Keeping the process calm and slow prevented frustration for both of us.

2. Simplifying Clothing Choices: Choosing clothes can be confusing for someone with dementia. We began laying out two simple outfit choices, limiting his options so he wouldn't feel overwhelmed. Choosing clothes with easy fastenings, like Velcro and elastic waistbands, allowed him to dress with minimal assistance. This small act of independence gave him pride and made him feel in control of his appearance.

3. Promoting Dignity: Personal care can be sensitive, especially when a loved one needs help with intimate tasks. We always approached these moments with respect and explained what we were doing as we went along. I'd often say things like, "Let's freshen up so you can feel comfortable," which helped him understand the goal without feeling embarrassed. Maintaining dignity was always our priority, even in the simplest acts of care.

Helping my dad with his hygiene and dressing routine gave him a sense of autonomy, and it reminded us to be patient and understanding. These small acts of daily care became ways to preserve his independence while providing the support he needed.

Managing Medications

Managing medications can become a complicated part of caregiving, especially when multiple prescriptions are involved. Creating a system for medication management helped ensure that my dad received the right doses at the right times, minimizing risks and keeping his treatment on track.

1. Organizing Medications: We used a pill organizer with labeled compartments for each day of the week and specific times of day. This tool simplified the process and made it easy for us to see if a dose had been missed. Keeping his medications in a single, easily accessible place also helped avoid confusion.

2. Setting Reminders: To ensure my dad took his medications on time, we set reminders on our phones. Alarms went off each time he needed his medicine, creating a reliable system for both us and him. This consistency made him feel more comfortable, as he could predict the routine of taking his pills without feeling rushed or confused.

3. Tracking Side Effects: Monitoring for side effects was an essential part of his medication routine. We kept a notebook where we'd note

any unusual symptoms, like dizziness or appetite changes, and discussed these with his doctor. By tracking his reactions, we could adjust the medications if needed, ensuring he received safe, effective care.

A structured approach to medication management kept my dad's health stable, and the consistency of the routine helped him feel secure in his daily life. With a system in place, we were able to focus more on enjoying quality time together without the constant worry of managing his pills.

Food and Nutrition

Nutrition plays a crucial role in supporting brain health and maintaining physical well-being. People with dementia may experience appetite loss, difficulty eating, or forgetfulness around meals. Creating a balanced diet with familiar foods and keeping an eye on hydration became essential parts of our caregiving routine.

1. Balanced Meals with Familiar Foods: Serving balanced meals that included proteins, whole grains, and vegetables helped keep my dad's energy steady. We found that familiar foods

from his past often appealed to him more, so we'd include dishes he loved, like soups or soft foods that were easy for him to chew and digest. Keeping meals simple and visually appealing encouraged him to eat without feeling overwhelmed.

2. Handling Appetite Loss: Over time, my dad's appetite began to decline, and he would sometimes leave his meals unfinished. We adapted by offering smaller, more frequent meals and snacks rather than large meals. Foods high in healthy fats, like avocados and nuts, provided more calories without requiring a large portion. Sometimes, a small bowl of his favorite pudding or a smoothie would do the trick when he wasn't up for a full meal.

3. Staying Hydrated: Dehydration is common in dementia because people may forget to drink water. To make sure he stayed hydrated, we kept a water bottle within his reach and set reminders throughout the day. We also offered fruits high in water content, like oranges and watermelon, to supplement his fluid intake. These small efforts helped us avoid dehydration, which can quickly impact mood and cognition.

Focusing on his nutrition and hydration needs became a way to support his health and well-being. Adapting to his changing tastes and needs showed us the importance of flexibility and creativity in caregiving.

If you are enjoying this book, and is helping you navigate your journey, I'd love to hear your honest review, it helps others find it too. Please take a moment and drop your review.

Share it with friends, family, or anyone who might benefit. And don't miss my other books designed to inspire and uplift your journey.
Your support means everything. Thank you!

Incontinence and Toileting Care

Incontinence is common in the later stages of dementia and can be a sensitive and challenging aspect of caregiving. Managing incontinence with dignity, empathy, and practical solutions helped us keep my dad comfortable and maintained his sense of self-respect.

1. Establishing a Bathroom Routine: Regular bathroom visits reduced accidents and maintained my dad's dignity. We would encourage him to use the bathroom every two hours, especially after meals and before bedtime. Sticking to this routine helped him feel more secure and lowered the risk of accidents.

2. Using Incontinence Products: We gradually introduced incontinence products, like protective underwear, when it became necessary. These products allowed him to move around comfortably without fear of embarrassment. We selected items that were discreet and comfortable, emphasizing that they were simply there to keep him comfortable, not to change his identity.

3. Maintaining Cleanliness with Respect: Helping with toileting requires sensitivity. We would always explain what we were doing and offer assistance gently, respecting his dignity throughout the process. Our focus was on his comfort and preserving his privacy. Using soft wipes and protective creams helped prevent skin irritation and made the routine as gentle as possible.

Managing incontinence was one of the more challenging aspects of caregiving, but we approached it with respect and patience. It became a way to show compassion and care for him in a time of vulnerability.

Each of these daily caregiving essentials helped us support my dad's well-being, independence, and dignity.

CHAPTER 6

Communication and Behavioral Management

Communication is one of the most challenging aspects of caring for someone with dementia, as the disease gradually impacts how a person thinks, understands, and interacts with others. Along with changes in communication, behavioral issues often arise, including agitation, wandering, and confusion. These behaviors can be distressing, but with patience and effective techniques, caregivers can create a calmer, more understanding environment for their loved ones. Here, I'll share the strategies and insights we developed while caring for my dad, along with ways to manage common dementia-related behaviors.

Effective Communication Techniques

Effective communication becomes more challenging as dementia progresses, but certain techniques can help make interactions more meaningful and reduce frustration for both caregiver and loved one.

- ***Using Clear, Simple Language:*** Dementia affects a person's ability to process complex language, so it's essential to use short, simple sentences. When speaking to my dad, I found it helpful to break down instructions into single steps. Instead of saying, "Let's get you dressed, brush your teeth, and then we'll have breakfast," I would say, "First, let's put on your shirt." This approach made it easier for him to understand and respond.

- ***Maintaining Eye Contact:*** Making eye contact helped us connect with my dad on a deeper level. By looking directly at him, I was able to capture his attention and convey that I was there, focused on him alone. Eye contact made him feel respected and seen, and it encouraged him to engage with me even when he seemed lost in thought.

- ***Practicing Active Listening:*** People with dementia often feel frustrated when they can't express themselves, so I learned the importance of truly listening. Giving my dad time to find his words and nodding along showed him that his thoughts mattered. Sometimes, he would pause mid-sentence, struggling to finish, and I would gently prompt him by repeating part of his thought. This reassured him that I was patient and there to listen, even if he couldn't find the words.

These communication techniques reduced misunderstandings and helped us maintain a strong connection. Though the words were sometimes few, we were still able to share meaningful moments.

Understanding Behavioral Changes

As dementia progresses, behavioral changes like agitation, aggression, repetitive actions, and wandering are common. These behaviors may seem random, but they often stem from unmet needs, confusion, or fear.

- *Agitation and Aggression*: Dementia can make it difficult for a person to express their emotions, leading to sudden agitation or aggression. When my dad became irritable, we often realized he was reacting to something in his environment. It might have been a loud noise, a physical discomfort, or simply feeling overwhelmed. To calm him, we learned to gently ask questions like, "Are you feeling uncomfortable?" or "Is something bothering you?" We found that removing him from a noisy room or playing soft music could often calm his mood.

- **Repetitive Actions:** Repetition, such as asking the same question multiple times, is common in dementia and can be frustrating for caregivers. I learned that my dad's repetitive questions often came from a need for reassurance. For example, he'd frequently ask, "When's dinner?" We would respond with the same calm answer each time, knowing that it was the reassurance, not the answer, that he needed. Creating visual reminders, like a note on the fridge with meal times, also helped reduce his anxiety about these routines.

- **Wandering**: Wandering can be particularly concerning, as it may lead to dangerous situations if a loved one becomes lost. My dad would sometimes leave the house, believing he needed to go to work or visit an old friend. We installed door alarms that would alert us if he left and made sure he wore an ID bracelet with his information. Additionally, we gently redirected him when he tried to go outside, saying things like, *"It's almost time for lunch. Let's get ready to eat together first."* This approach helped him refocus without feeling restricted.

There was a time he wandered to the store of our neighbour, Sammy gave him some snacks and he ate and was having a good time with her. At first my thought was to gently bring him home, but I heard his laughter with her and I just stayed back while listening to their conversation. All the while he spoke so well and his eyes were bright with happiness all over. For those few minutes he spent there, I saw the version of my dad I knew before.

Understanding these behaviors and their potential triggers helped us create a more supportive and responsive environment, keeping my dad safe while respecting his autonomy.

Managing Sundowning and Sleep Disturbances

Sundowning is a phenomenon in which people with dementia experience increased confusion, agitation, or restlessness in the late afternoon or evening. This can lead to sleep disturbances and make nighttime a challenging period for caregivers.

- ***Creating a Calm Environment:*** As evening approached, we dimmed the lights, reduced noise, and created a soothing environment. Bright lights or sudden sounds seemed to trigger anxiety for my dad, so we avoided watching loud TV shows or having busy conversations in the evening. Instead, we played calming music and focused on quiet activities, like reading or looking through photo albums together.

- ***Establishing a Bedtime Routine:*** A consistent bedtime routine can help reduce confusion and ease the transition to sleep. Every night, we followed the same sequence: turning off lights, brushing his teeth, and talking softly as he got ready for bed. We often read a few pages of his favorite book or sat together quietly until he felt relaxed. This familiar routine signaled to his mind that it was time to rest, which made a noticeable difference in his sleep quality.

- ***Using Calming Techniques***: When my dad became restless, we found that gentle hand massages or a warm cup of chamomile tea could calm him down. Touch, in particular, seemed to ease his anxiety and remind him that he was safe. When he was particularly agitated, I'd sit with him, hold his hand, and reassure him softly, which helped him settle.

By creating a peaceful evening environment and following a routine, we managed to reduce my dad's restlessness and improve his sleep. Sundowning can be challenging, but calming techniques helped us make the nights more restful for him and less stressful for us.

Coping with Hallucinations and Delusions

Hallucinations and delusions are not uncommon in dementia, especially as the disease progresses. Hallucinations involve seeing or hearing things that aren't there, while delusions are false beliefs, like thinking people are stealing from them. Responding to these symptoms with calm understanding can prevent escalation.

- ***Validating Their Feelings***: My dad sometimes saw things that weren't there, like a cat in the corner of the room or people outside the window. Rather than contradicting him, which only made him more upset, we acknowledged his experience. I would say, "I see you're looking at something. Is it the cat you're thinking of?" He remained composed and respected his view by having his sentiments validated without contributing to the illusion.

- ***Gently Redirecting***: When my dad believed someone was taking his belongings, we calmly reassured him by showing him where his items were.

Sometimes, he would accuse us of moving things, but instead of arguing, we'd say, *"Let's look together and see if we can find it."* Redirecting his focus to a new activity or conversation also helped distract him from his delusion without making him feel dismissed.

- ***Reducing Environmental Triggers***: We found that certain things—like shadows, reflections, or even clutter—could trigger my dad's hallucinations. Closing blinds in the evening or removing reflective surfaces reduced these triggers and made him feel more at ease. We learned that small adjustments to the environment could have a big impact on his sense of security.

Coping with hallucinations and delusions requires patience and creativity. By validating his feelings and gently redirecting his focus, we helped him feel understood and reassured.

De-escalation Strategies

Emotional outbursts, including anger, crying, or frustration, can be triggered by confusion, fear, or a simple miscommunication. Knowing how to de-escalate these moments is crucial for both the caregiver and the person with dementia.

- ***Staying Calm and Composed:*** Remaining calm was the most effective way to de-escalate my dad's outbursts. When he became upset, raising my voice or showing frustration only made things worse. Rather, I discovered how to inhale deeply, talk quietly, and comfort him. My calm demeanor helped him mirror that calmness, allowing him to feel safe and reducing his distress.

- ***Using Soothing Language***: Gentle, reassuring phrases worked wonders during his moments of agitation. When my dad was particularly distressed, I'd say things like, *"I'm here with you,"* or *"Everything is okay."* These simple phrases reminded him that he wasn't alone and that he was safe. Over time, we noticed he became more receptive to these calming words.

- ***Engaging in Distraction Techniques:*** Distraction was a valuable tool in diffusing tension. If my dad became upset over a small issue, we'd gently shift his focus by offering him a snack, turning on soft music, or suggesting a short walk. This redirection allowed him to move past the frustration without needing to dwell on it.

- **Recognizing Triggers:** We began to recognize patterns in his outbursts. For example, my dad often became frustrated during transitions, like moving from one room to another or changing clothes. We planned these moments carefully, giving him extra time and preparing him in advance, which helped him feel more in control and reduced his agitation.

By incorporating these communication and behavioral management techniques into our daily caregiving, we created a more peaceful and supportive environment for my dad. Understanding the changes in his behavior and learning to respond with patience allowed us to provide the best care possible, even on challenging days.

CHAPTER 7

Physical and Cognitive Health Management

How can I keep my loved one with dementia healthy and engaged? What activities are safe, and how can I help them feel mentally stimulated? These are common questions you must have asked yourself, and addressing both physical and cognitive health is essential. Physical health management promotes strength, mobility, and safety, while cognitive stimulation helps preserve memory and focus, offering moments of joy and connection. In our journey with my dad, these daily activities became a way to care for him holistically, nurturing both his body and mind.

Exercise and Mobility

Exercise may look different for people with dementia, but it remains an essential part of care. Gentle movement supports muscle strength, coordination, and mental well-being. For my dad, physical activity was a great way to start the day, helping him feel more energized and less anxious.

1. **Gentle Exercises**: Simple exercises like walking, stretching, and light arm and leg movements provided a safe way for my dad to stay active. Each morning, we'd walk around the block or even just around the house if the weather was bad. These short walks were beneficial for both his physical and mental health, and it was a time when we could talk and connect in a calm setting.

2. **Fall Prevention**: Balance issues are common in dementia, so reducing the risk of falls was one of our top priorities. We cleared pathways, removed rugs, and added non-slip mats in the bathroom. We also encouraged my dad to use handrails and stable furniture for support. One of the most effective measures was providing him with sturdy, well-fitted shoes that gave him extra stability.

3. **Using Mobility Aids:** As his dementia progressed, my dad needed more physical support. Introducing a walker allowed him to continue moving around with more confidence and independence. While he was hesitant at first, we reassured him that the walker was there to keep him safe, not to limit him. Over time, he adapted to using it, and it became part of his daily routine.

Cognitive Stimulation Activities

Cognitive stimulation is crucial for keeping the mind engaged. While dementia impacts memory and processing, familiar activities can help slow cognitive decline and provide a sense of accomplishment.

1. ***Puzzles and Memory Games:*** My dad loved puzzles, so we started with simple ones—like large-piece jigsaw puzzles. These exercises were mentally stimulating and satisfying for him, and they gave us time to sit together and enjoy each other's company. Memory games, like matching pictures or short word games, also helped him exercise his mind without feeling overwhelmed.

If you are enjoying this book, and it is helping you navigate your journey, I'd love to hear your honest review, it helps others find it too . Share it with friends, family, or anyone who might benefit.

And don't miss my other books designed to inspire and uplift your journey. They are for kids but they can as well help your loved ones. They are listed at the end of the book.
Thank you for your support.

2. **Reading Familiar Books**: While reading new material became challenging, revisiting familiar stories brought comfort. We often read his favorite short stories and poems together, ones he had known for years. Sometimes, he'd recall a line or phrase, and seeing his face light up in recognition was priceless. These moments reminded us that even though he was losing his short-term memory, his love for certain stories remained.

3. **Art and Creative Expression**: Art became a wonderful outlet for my dad. We'd set up simple art projects with markers, colored pencils, or even clay. Even if his drawings were abstract, the act of creating gave him a sense of purpose and joy. Art allowed him to express emotions he couldn't put into words, and it was a relaxing activity we could enjoy together.

Incorporating cognitive stimulation into his daily routine gave my dad moments of joy and preserved parts of his personality. These activities offered him dignity and a sense of accomplishment, even as his memory faded.

Mental Health Care

Mental health care is essential in dementia, as people often experience depression, anxiety, and frustration due to changes in memory and behavior. Recognizing these signs early can improve quality of life and prevent unnecessary suffering.

1. ***Identifying Depression:*** Depression is common in dementia, but its symptoms can be subtle. My dad became withdrawn and less interested in activities he once loved. He seemed quieter, spending more time looking out the window than talking with us. Recognizing this shift, we spoke to his doctor, who recommended adjustments in his routine and gentle encouragement to participate in daily activities.

2. ***Managing Anxiety:*** My dad sometimes felt anxious, especially in unfamiliar settings or around loud noises. His anxiety would show up as restlessness, like pacing or wringing his hands. To help him feel grounded, we kept his surroundings calm and familiar. Soft background music, gentle lighting, and our reassuring presence helped soothe his nerves.

3. ***Providing Emotional Reassurance***: Simple gestures like holding his hand, listening to his worries, or even sitting quietly together brought comfort. We tried to validate his emotions by saying things like, "I understand it's a bit confusing," rather than dismissing his feelings. Reassurance went a long way in helping him feel safe.

Supporting his mental health helped reduce his anxiety and brought him moments of calm and contentment. Small changes in routine and a focus on his emotional needs had a positive impact on his overall well-being.

Monitoring Health Conditions

People with dementia may have other health conditions, such as diabetes or high blood pressure, which require careful management. Overseeing these conditions became a key part of my dad's daily care.

1. ***Monitoring Blood Sugar Levels***: My dad had diabetes, so keeping his blood sugar under control was essential. We kept a schedule for his blood sugar checks, making sure to monitor it before meals and after any physical activity. Consistency was important,

and the routine of testing his blood sugar became a part of our daily ritual.

2. ***Managing Blood Pressure***: Monitoring blood pressure helped us prevent complications and keep his overall health stable. We had a home blood pressure monitor that we used once or twice a week. These regular check-ins became especially important when he was on new medications or when his behavior seemed unusually agitated.

3. ***Coordinating with Healthcare Providers:*** Communication with his doctors was essential for managing his other health conditions. Regular check-ups allowed us to discuss his blood sugar and blood pressure, adjust medications, and address any side effects. His doctors appreciated that we kept detailed notes on his symptoms, and it helped them make informed decisions about his care.

By monitoring his health conditions and communicating with his healthcare team, we helped maintain his physical health. This proactive care allowed us to prevent issues and focus on creating a stable, comfortable routine for him.

Recognizing and Managing Pain

People with dementia may not always be able to communicate their pain verbally, which can lead to discomfort and agitation. Understanding nonverbal cues became essential in recognizing when my dad was in pain.

1. **Observing Nonverbal Cues:** When my dad was uncomfortable, he often showed it through body language rather than words. He'd grimace, hold a certain part of his body, or appear more restless than usual. These subtle cues were signs that something was bothering him, even if he couldn't say it out loud. We learned to watch for these signs, knowing they could indicate physical discomfort.

2. **Asking Simple Questions**: To check if he was in pain, we'd ask simple questions like, *"Does your arm hurt?"* or *"Are you feeling okay here?"* This allowed him to give a basic yes or no answer without the pressure of explaining. When he nodded or pointed, it helped us narrow down the issue and take action, like adjusting his seating or applying a warm compress to relieve aches.

3. **Providing Gentle Comfort Measures**: Simple pain-relief strategies, like a warm blanket, gentle massages, or a change in seating position, often eased his discomfort. If he seemed more relaxed afterward, we knew we were on the right track. This hands-on approach helped us address his needs while reducing his stress.

Understanding and addressing his pain helped prevent emotional distress and contributed to his overall sense of well-being. Even when he couldn't say what hurt, our careful observation allowed us to respond with empathy and make sure he was as comfortable as possible.

By focusing on his physical health, cognitive engagement, and emotional needs, we were able to make each day a little brighter, preserving our connection even as dementia progressed.

CHAPTER 8

Legal and Financial Planning

When dementia enters your life, legal and financial planning becomes an essential part of caregiving. It's a way to safeguard the future and provide a sense of security for both the person with dementia and their family. This chapter will explore the key areas in legal and financial planning, from preparing crucial documents to ensuring the rights and dignity of your loved one. When we started this process for my dad, it was both emotional and empowering. Knowing that his wishes were in place gave us a sense of peace, allowing us to focus more on being present with him.

Legal Documents to Prepare

One of the first steps in planning for dementia care is creating legal documents that clearly outline a loved one's preferences and provide decision-making authority if they're unable to make those decisions independently. These documents prevent confusion and ensure that their wishes are honored.

1. **Power of Attorney (POA)**: A legal document that grants someone (the "agent") the ability to make financial choices on behalf of another (the "principal") is a power of attorney (POA). This can cover everything from paying bills to managing bank accounts and investments. My dad wanted me to handle his finances when he could no longer manage them, so we drafted a power of attorney early on. Setting it up early ensured that he had a say in who managed his finances, and it made handling his affairs smoother as the disease progressed.

2. **Living Will**: A living will is a document that states a person's wishes regarding medical treatments they do or do not want, especially at the end of life. It includes directives on life-support measures, resuscitation, and pain management. Although it was hard to discuss these topics, my dad was clear about wanting a natural end-of-life experience without aggressive medical intervention. Having his living will in place was invaluable to us later, as we knew we were honoring his desires.

3. **Health Care Proxy:** A healthcare proxy designates someone to make healthcare decisions if a person becomes unable to make

them independently. My dad chose my sister for this role, as she had a strong understanding of his values and healthcare preferences. We felt relief knowing that someone close to him would make choices aligned with his wishes, and it prevented disagreements among family members.

Preparing these documents early gave my dad control over his future. It was a powerful experience for him, allowing him to express his choices while he still could, and it gave us a solid foundation to respect those choices as his dementia progressed.

Financial Planning for Long-Term Care

The cost of long-term dementia care can be overwhelming, so financial planning is essential to ensure resources are used wisely and the necessary care is accessible. From budgeting to exploring government programs, we had to learn a lot about financial planning to make sure my dad's needs were met.

1. ***Budgeting for Care Costs***: Long-term care can be expensive, whether at home, in an assisted living facility, or in a nursing home.

We began by creating a budget that covered all expected costs, including home modifications, medical supplies, and potential costs for in-home care assistance. Writing down all possible expenses helped us see what was realistic and adjust other areas of the budget to accommodate care.

2. ***Insurance Options:*** Long-term care insurance can cover some dementia care expenses, like nursing home care, in-home support, or adult day programs. Unfortunately, my dad didn't have long-term care insurance, but we explored his existing health insurance policy to see what services were covered. Some insurance policies provide limited coverage for certain in-home services, which helped reduce out-of-pocket expenses.

3. ***Government Programs:*** Government programs like Medicaid can be a lifeline for dementia care. Medicaid offers assistance for low-income individuals who need long-term care but have limited resources. While my dad didn't qualify for Medicaid, we found that several state-level programs provided financial aid for in-home support and respite care. Exploring these options is worth the time, as they can ease the financial burden significantly.

4. **_Veterans' Benefits_**: If your loved one is a veteran, they may qualify for aid through the Department of Veterans Affairs (VA). VA benefits can cover in-home care, adult day programs, or nursing home care. My dad wasn't a veteran, but a friend of ours found great support for their family through these benefits, which can make a big difference for eligible families.

This financial planning process helped us feel prepared for the future. By considering all options and creating a detailed budget, we could provide my dad with high-quality care while managing resources responsibly.

Rights of the Person with Dementia

People with dementia have the same rights to dignity, respect, and autonomy as anyone else. However, dementia can put these rights at risk, as caregivers and family members may unintentionally overlook their preferences or push them aside for convenience.

1. **_Preserving Dignity_**: One of the most fundamental rights is the right to be treated with dignity. Even as my dad's memory and

behavior changed, we ensured he was always spoken to with respect. Small gestures, like asking for his input on daily activities or treating him with patience, reinforced his dignity and reminded us that he was still the same person.

2. **_Protecting Privacy:_** As dementia progresses, a person may need more physical assistance, which can impact their privacy. We always made sure to explain what we were doing before assisting my dad with personal care tasks and respected his modesty whenever possible. Preserving his privacy maintained his sense of self-respect, which was crucial for his emotional well-being.

3. **_Maintaining Autonomy_**: Autonomy, or the right to make decisions about one's own life, is also essential. Even as his dementia worsened, we encouraged my dad to make choices, like what he wanted to wear or what he'd like for lunch. This involvement reminded him that he still had a voice in his care. Recognizing his rights helped us provide care that was both respectful and compassionate.

Ensuring the rights of people with dementia is not only about legal obligations but also about treating them with the respect they deserve. By prioritizing dignity, privacy, and autonomy, we were able to honor my dad's identity and values.

Making Decisions Together

Including the person with dementia in planning decisions is vital, as it reinforces their role in their own life. Though decision-making abilities may change, involving them early ensures their preferences are known and respected.

1. ***Discussing Preferences Early On:*** When my dad was first diagnosed, we made a point to talk about his preferences for future care. He shared his wish to stay at home as long as possible and specified which family members he'd feel comfortable with for certain tasks. This early conversation helped us create a plan that aligned with his wishes, and he felt more secure knowing his voice was heard.

2. ***Simplifying Decisions:*** As dementia progresses, making complex decisions becomes challenging, so we started simplifying choices. Instead of asking open-ended questions, we'd offer limited options, like "Do you want the

blue shirt or the red one?" With this method, my dad was able to take part in decision-making without feeling overwhelmed. Even these small choices helped him feel in control of his day.

3. ***Involving Him in Financial Planning***: While he could still understand, we went over the basics of financial planning together. My dad appreciated being involved and knowing that his hard-earned savings would go toward his care. By sharing these plans, we made sure he felt valued and aware of how his future needs would be managed.

Involving the person with dementia in their own planning reinforces their autonomy and creates a sense of partnership in care. These conversations are not only practical but also emotionally rewarding, providing peace of mind for everyone involved.

Guardianship and Conservatorship

Guardianship and conservatorship are legal arrangements in which a court appoints someone to make decisions on behalf of a person who can no longer manage their own affairs. These roles are sometimes necessary for individuals with advanced dementia when other legal measures are insufficient.

1. **What is Guardianship?** Through guardianship, a court designates a person (the "guardian") to make choices regarding a person's personal and medical care on their behalf if they are incapable of doing so themselves. Guardianship can cover decisions like where the person will live, what care they will receive, and how their daily needs will be managed. This can be especially helpful if there are disagreements among family members or if a person's condition has declined to the point where they cannot communicate.

2. *Understanding Conservatorship:* Conservatorship is specifically associated with financial issues. A conservator manages finances, handles bills, and oversees property on behalf of the individual. This role is important when someone is unable to manage their finances but hasn't designated a power of attorney. It can help ensure that the person's resources are protected and used appropriately for their care.

3. **When Guardianship or Conservatorship is Necessary:** We didn't

require guardianship for my dad, as his power of attorney and healthcare proxy were in place early. However, for families where these documents aren't completed in time, guardianship or conservatorship may become necessary. Since these arrangements entail a loss of personal autonomy, they ought to be reserved for extreme circumstances. A court will review the person's condition and determine if such measures are necessary, and the guardian or conservator must report to the court periodically.

4. **Respecting the Person's Rights**: Even with guardianship or conservatorship, it's essential to respect the person's dignity. Guardians should involve their loved one in decisions as much as possible, ensuring that their wishes and values guide each choice. These roles are about protection, not control, and should be approached with empathy.

Understanding guardianship and conservatorship helped us realize how important it was to prepare legal documents early. Knowing these options allowed us to make informed choices that respected my dad's independence.

A Caregiver's Guide for Dementia and Alzheimer's Disease

Legal and financial planning can seem daunting, but each step creates a foundation for compassionate, respectful care. For us, making these plans early was like building a safety net that let us focus on my dad's needs and well-being rather than worrying about logistics. By ensuring his wishes were in place and protecting his rights, we could honor him in a way that truly reflected his values, giving us all peace and purpose as we navigated the journey together.

If you are enjoying this book, and it is helping you navigate your journey, I'd love to hear your honest review, it helps others find it too . Share it with friends, family, or anyone who might benefit. And don't miss my other books designed to inspire and uplift your journey.

Your support means everything. Thank you!

CHAPTER 9

Self-Care and Support for Caregivers

One night, after a long day of caring for my dad, I remember finally sitting down, exhausted and emotionally drained. I hadn't slept well in days, and my back ached from helping him move around the house. At that moment, I realized that I was so focused on his needs that I had completely neglected my own. Like so many caregivers, I found myself in a constant state of "just one more thing" until I had nothing left to give. I realized I couldn't keep caring for him effectively unless I took time to care for myself.

But how do you make time for yourself when caregiving already consumes so much energy and attention? This is a question almost every caregiver wrestles with. The answer lies in understanding that taking care of yourself is not selfish; it's necessary. If we're constantly running on empty, our ability to provide compassionate and effective care diminishes. In this section, we'll explore essential practices for caregiver self-care, from recognizing burnout to finding practical ways to recharge.

The Importance of Self-Care

Caregiving is a full-time role that requires physical, mental, and emotional strength. However, many caregivers feel guilty about taking breaks, worrying that any time spent away from caregiving is time lost. The truth is that self-care is crucial, and neglecting it can lead to serious health issues, including depression, anxiety, and physical exhaustion.

1. ***Sustaining Long-Term Care***: When I realized I was running on empty, it became clear that I couldn't support my dad if I wasn't also taking care of myself. Caring for someone with dementia can be a long journey, and to go the distance, we need to maintain our own strength. By prioritizing sleep, balanced meals, and regular checkups, I could stay healthier and more alert, ready to be there for him.

2. ***Preventing Compassion Fatigue:*** Compassion fatigue is common among caregivers who pour all their energy into caring for someone else. Over time, this can cause emotional numbness, where you're physically

present but emotionally distant. Self-care helps keep compassion alive, allowing caregivers to feel refreshed and ready to connect. Small moments of self-care—whether it's taking a short walk or listening to music—allowed me to approach caregiving with renewed patience and empathy.

Self-care is not an indulgence; it's a vital part of being able to provide quality care. By making our well-being a priority, we not only take better care of ourselves but also create a healthier caregiving environment.

Identifying Caregiver Burnout

Caregiver burnout is a state of physical, mental, and emotional exhaustion that can result from the relentless demands of caregiving. Burnout doesn't happen overnight; it builds gradually, often going unnoticed until it becomes overwhelming.

1. **Physical Signs:** Exhaustion, frequent illness, and sleep problems are common physical signs of burnout. I remember constantly catching colds and having lingering aches and pains, signs that my body was under stress. When you're constantly on alert and

focused on someone else's needs, your body misses the chance to recover, which weakens your immune system and resilience.

2. **Emotional Signs:** Caregiver burnout can also manifest as irritability, anxiety, and a sense of hopelessness. At one point, I found myself feeling resentful and frustrated over small things, a sign that I was emotionally drained. Recognizing these feelings was hard, as I didn't want to admit I was struggling, but acknowledging them was the first step toward finding balance.

3. **Social Withdrawal**: Burnout often leads caregivers to withdraw from friends, family, and activities they once enjoyed. I found myself turning down invitations, feeling too tired or emotionally drained to socialize. Over time, this isolation intensified feelings of loneliness and made caregiving even harder. Understanding that these were signs of burnout helped me realize the importance of staying connected with others.

Recognizing these symptoms of burnout is crucial, as it will allow you to take steps toward self-care before reaching a breaking point. By addressing burnout early, we can avoid long-term physical and emotional damage and continue caring with love and patience.

Stress Management Techniques

Managing stress is essential for you as a caregiver, as chronic stress can quickly lead to burnout. Stress management techniques can help bring calm to difficult moments and create space to process emotions.

1. **Mindfulness**: Practicing mindfulness involves staying present in the moment without judgment. I found that taking even five minutes each day to focus on my breathing and observe my thoughts helped me clear my mind. Whether I was helping my dad with his meals or taking him for a walk, practicing mindfulness helped me stay calm and centered, allowing me to be more patient.

2. **Deep Breathing**: Deep breathing exercises are a quick and effective way to reduce stress. When my dad would become agitated, I'd often feel my own anxiety rise. In those moments, I'd take a few slow, deep breaths, focusing on inhaling and exhaling. This simple exercise helped me stay grounded, allowing me to

respond to him with a calm tone rather than with frustration.

3. **Journaling**: Journaling became an outlet for expressing emotions that were hard to share with others. Writing down my thoughts helped me process the highs and lows of caregiving. Sometimes I'd jot down positive memories or small victories, like a day when he smiled at an old memory. Other times, I'd write about the challenges. Reflecting on these entries allowed me to recognize patterns in my own emotions, helping me understand my journey as a caregiver.

Stress management doesn't require a lot of time; even small practices can have a significant impact. By integrating these techniques into my day, I was able to release tension and find moments of peace, even in difficult times.

Finding Time for Yourself

Finding time for yourself as a caregiver may seem impossible, but even small breaks can be incredibly restorative. Taking time to rest or pursue personal interests can prevent burnout and keep you engaged in caregiving.

1. ***Using Respite Care:*** Respite care provides temporary relief for caregivers by allowing someone else to care for your loved one. We arranged for my dad to attend an adult day program a few times a week, where he could participate in activities and socialize. This gave us a few hours to recharge, run errands, or simply take a breather. Knowing he was safe and engaged made it easier to relax and enjoy the time for ourselves.

2. ***Delegating Tasks:*** Caregiving is often a team effort, and sharing responsibilities can make a big difference. I learned to accept help from family members and close friends, who would sit with my dad, bring over meals, or handle small tasks. Delegating even a few duties provided some mental space, and it reminded me that I didn't have to carry the load alone.

3. ***Scheduling Personal Time***: Setting aside time for yourself—even if it's just 20 minutes—can provide valuable relief. I started scheduling small breaks into my day, where I'd read a book, take a walk, or call a friend. These short, intentional breaks helped me recharge, allowing me to return to caregiving with a fresh perspective and renewed patience.

Your own well-being is an investment when you take time for yourself. These breaks aren't just about "escaping" caregiving; they're about restoring your energy so you can continue to provide care from a place of compassion and strength.

Counseling and Support Groups

Caregiving can feel isolating, but connecting with others who understand the experience can be a powerful source of comfort and strength. Counseling and support groups provide a safe space to share challenges, gain new insights, and receive emotional support.

1. ***Individual Counseling:*** Talking to a counselor gave me a safe space to express emotions that were sometimes hard to share with family. Counseling helped me process feelings of guilt, frustration, and sadness, allowing me to approach caregiving with a clearer mind and a lighter heart. My counselor also taught me coping strategies that I could use in moments of stress, which improved my overall resilience.

2. Support Groups: Attending a support group was one of the most helpful steps I took as a

caregiver. Being in a room with people who truly understood the highs and lows of dementia care made me feel less alone. Hearing others' stories provided a new perspective, and sometimes a simple piece of advice from another caregiver would make my day-to-day routine easier. I realized that my struggles were shared by many, which brought a sense of solidarity and strength.

3. **Online Communities**: If in-person support isn't available, online communities can provide valuable connections. I joined an online group for caregivers, where people shared advice, resources, and encouragement. Having access to this community anytime—whether during a late-night worry or a quiet moment—was invaluable. These groups offered the same compassion and support as an in-person group, with the convenience of connecting from home.

Emotional support is vital in caregiving, and sharing experiences can be both comforting and enlightening. Support groups and counseling provided me with tools, strength, and a community, reminding me that I didn't have to navigate this journey alone.

In the end, caring for yourself isn't just about your own well-being; it's about being able to care for your loved one with a steady heart and a clear mind. Each small act of self-care made me a better caregiver for my dad, allowing me to show up fully, day after day, with patience and compassion.

CHAPTER 10

Advanced and End-of-Life Care

As dementia progresses into its advanced stages, caregiving takes on a new level of complexity. The needs of the person with dementia change, often requiring around-the-clock care and new considerations for their physical, emotional, and spiritual comfort. These moments, while incredibly difficult, can also be profoundly meaningful. In caring for my dad through his final days, our family faced many challenges, but we also found strength, love, and deep connection. This chapter covers the essential aspects of advanced and end-of-life care, from preparing for full-time care to finding ways to honor and remember a loved one's life.

Transitioning to Full-Time Care

Transitioning to full-time care is a significant step, one that requires careful planning, open discussions with family, and sometimes professional support. Full-time care means being available day and night, as advanced dementia often brings changes in sleeping patterns, physical abilities, and communication.

1. **Creating a Structured Environment**: For my dad, we found that having a highly structured environment helped him feel more secure. We set up consistent routines for meals, personal care, and quiet times. As dementia progressed, these routines gave him a sense of predictability, even when he could no longer communicate it. This structured approach also allowed our family to share caregiving responsibilities more smoothly.

2. **Adjusting the Home for Safety**: Safety becomes increasingly important as dementia progresses. We made further modifications to our home, such as using bed rails, installing additional grab bars in the bathroom, and moving his bed close to a window to bring natural light into his space. These changes created a safe environment that minimized risks while providing him with a comforting place to rest.

3. **Accepting Outside Help:** Moving to full-time care can be overwhelming for families. Accepting help from home health aides or respite care providers allowed us to

manage the physical demands while ensuring my dad had the best possible care. The added support gave us time to recharge, which helped us stay emotionally connected to him instead of feeling consumed by the constant demands of caregiving.

Transitioning to full-time care was challenging, but it also strengthened our bond with him. We learned to cherish each moment, knowing that providing him with peace and comfort was the most important thing we could do.

Hospice and Palliative Care

As dementia advances, hospice and palliative care can play a critical role in providing comfort and support. Both focus on improving quality of life and managing symptoms, but hospice care is specifically for end-of-life, while palliative care can begin earlier, alongside other treatments.

1. Palliative Care: Palliative care focuses on relieving symptoms, managing pain, and addressing the emotional and psychological needs of the person with dementia. When my dad started experiencing more pain and restlessness, we added palliative care to his

treatment. This allowed us to work with a team of professionals dedicated to keeping him comfortable, without the pressure of hospital visits or intense interventions.

2. Hospice Care: Hospice care is generally introduced when a doctor believes a person has six months or less to live. For my dad, hospice meant we could focus entirely on his comfort and dignity. The hospice team provided medications to ease his pain, supported our family emotionally, and helped us understand what to expect as he neared the end of his journey. Having this support allowed us to spend quality time with him, focused on love and peace rather than procedures and treatments.

3. Holistic Comfort: Both palliative and hospice care look beyond physical symptoms to address emotional and spiritual well-being. Simple comforts, like his favorite music, soft lighting, and family photos, became central to his care. These small touches created an atmosphere of calm and familiarity, which seemed to ease his mind and brought us closer together in his final days.

> *These were the worst times of my life, before dementia my dad and I shared a lot in common. We were best of friends. I promised him lots of things and he did too, but all of a sudden he had a few months to live. I didn't know which one to accept if it was the news of him having dementia or having a few months to live. I acted all strong and tough but I was breaking inside.*

Hospice and palliative care taught us to focus on the quality of his remaining time. These services allowed us to share gentle, memorable moments that honored his life, even as it was drawing to a close.

Emotional and Spiritual Support

End-of-life care involves more than simply symptom management; it also involves providing spiritual and emotional support. Honoring a person's beliefs, values, and memories can bring comfort and help them feel at peace with the life they've lived.

1. **Recognizing Spiritual Needs**: For my dad, spirituality had always been a personal

journey rather than one tied to a particular tradition. In his final weeks, we spent time reflecting on his life and the values he held dear. We'd often sit together, looking at photos or recalling stories from his childhood. This process was incredibly comforting for him, and it helped him feel connected to his past, his family, and his faith in something greater.

2. **Legacy-Building:** Legacy-building is a way to create lasting memories and honor the impact a loved one has had on others. As a family, we decided to gather stories from relatives and friends, creating a book of memories for him and future generations. We read these stories to him, which made him smile, and sometimes he'd add a few details of his own. This book became a precious gift for our family, preserving his voice and legacy.

3. **Offering Peaceful Moments**: Simple acts, like holding his hand or sitting in quiet companionship, became meaningful ways to provide emotional and spiritual support. Just being present with him in those moments of silence or speaking softly about shared memories helped ease his mind. These moments reminded us that love and

connection endure, even when words and memories fade.

> *I was always present and holding his hands because I didn't want him to leave but he still did.*

Emotional and spiritual support created a profound sense of peace in our family. It allowed us to honor his journey and provided him with comfort and meaning in his final days.

Family Grief and Support

Caring for a loved one with dementia is a unique experience, marked by a gradual form of grief as you witness changes in their personality and abilities. Preparing for the loss can help you find healthy ways to grieve and honor their memory.

1. **Anticipatory Grief:** Anticipatory grief is the sadness and loss we feel while a loved one is still alive but changing. With my dad, we had to come to terms with losing parts of him long before he passed. Acknowledging this grief,

rather than suppressing it, helped us process the emotions as they came, making the transition a bit gentler when he finally passed.

2. ***Finding Support for Grief:*** Grieving is not something that happens in isolation, and finding support was essential for our family. We leaned on each other, sharing memories and offering comfort. Support groups, whether in-person or online, provided a space to talk with others who understood the unique grief of dementia caregiving. Knowing we weren't alone helped ease the weight of the loss and allowed us to support each other.

I still don't know where I found the strength to write all these. The passing of my dad hit me badly. The fact that I was already missing him when he was still alive is very painful. Most times I told my family that I was going to visit some friends, I just found a corner to cry because I knew he was going and I couldn't do anything again.

---

3. ***Honoring Their Memory***: After my dad passed, we found small but meaningful ways to honor his memory. We held a quiet family

gathering, where each of us shared a story or a quality we loved about him. Later, we planted a tree in his honor—a living reminder of his presence in our lives. These acts of remembrance became healing rituals, allowing us to celebrate his life and keep his memory alive.

Preparing for grief allowed us to embrace the reality of loss with acceptance and love. Honoring my dad's memory became a source of strength, helping us remember that he would always be a part of our lives.

Whenever I see little children and their dads having a good time, the memories I had with my dad just click.

Legacy Planning and Bereavement

Legacy planning and bereavement are ways to reflect on a loved one's life, celebrate their contributions, and find closure. This process can bring comfort and help you carry forward the values and memories that defined them.

A Caregiver's Guide for Dementia and Alzheimer's Disease

1. **Legacy Planning:** Legacy planning can include creating a lasting tribute, such as a photo album, a memoir, or a donation to a cause they cared about. For my dad, we organized his belongings and preserved a few meaningful items—a pocket watch, his favorite hat, and a few handwritten letters. These keepsakes reminded us of the man he was, and they helped us feel connected to his spirit.

2. **Celebrating Their Life:** Celebrating a loved one's life can take many forms, from a simple family gathering to a formal memorial service. After my dad's passing, we hosted a celebration where family and friends shared stories, laughed, and remembered the special moments he brought to our lives. This celebration wasn't about mourning his death; it was about cherishing his life and the joy he had given us.

Up until now I still stay in my dad's room. I prefer it to mine, so I transferred my things there. Some people lock the door of their deceased loved ones, but I'm staying in my dad's room.

---

3. ***Finding Closure through Reflection:*** Bereavement is an ongoing process that takes time, reflection, and support. For me, writing about my dad—recalling our experiences and the lessons he taught—became a way to find closure. These reflections helped me accept the reality of his passing while holding onto the love and memories we shared.

> *My mom always says, " the death of a loved one is like a wound on the palm, you see the scars continually".*

Legacy planning and bereavement transformed our grief into a celebration of my dad's life. It allowed us to let go with peace and gratitude, knowing that his memory would live on in our hearts and in the stories we shared.

By focusing on comfort and finding ways to remember and celebrate a loved one's legacy, we can navigate this journey with grace. For our family, caring for my dad until the very end was an experience filled with both heartache and beauty. His memory lives on in each of us, a reminder that love endures beyond any goodbye. My dad passed away on the 28th of April, 2022.

CHAPTER 11

Real-Life Stories and Case Studies

How do caregivers find strength through the most difficult moments? Every caregiving journey has its challenges, but it's also filled with resilience, humor, and countless small victories. My journey with my dad taught me that caregivers are some of the most resilient people, finding strength, love, and even laughter in unexpected moments. In this chapter, I'll share stories from my own experience, along with lessons and memories from other caregivers who've walked similar paths. These stories serve as reminders that, while caregiving can be overwhelming, it's also deeply meaningful.

Caregivers Share How They've Coped and Found Strength
Resilience isn't something you have right from the beginning—it grows with each challenge and every moment of care. When my dad was first diagnosed, I was overwhelmed, thinking I wasn't strong enough to handle what lay ahead.

But over time, I learned that resilience often comes from simply showing up, day after day.

1. **The Small Steps Forward:** One caregiver I met at a support group shared how she coped with her mother's dementia by focusing on "small victories." She called it her *"one good thing"* practice. Each day, she'd find one positive thing to focus on, even if it was as small as her mom enjoying a cup of tea. Inspired by her, I started to look for "one good thing" every day with my dad. Some days, it was a shared smile or a gentle moment of recognition. Focusing on these small wins gave me strength and kept me going.

2. **Leaning on Support**: In the online community I was in another caregiver shared how she found strength in her family by letting them support her when she felt overwhelmed. Initially, she'd tried to handle all the caregiving on her own, but as her father's needs grew, she reached out for help from siblings and close friends. Following her example, I learned to lean on family, dividing tasks and finding comfort in the shared support. It taught me that resilience doesn't mean doing it all alone—it means knowing when to ask for help.

3. ***Acceptance and Adaptation:*** There was a point when I felt completely drained and questioned if I could continue caring for my dad as his condition worsened. At a support meeting, an older caregiver told me, *"You'll find a way through this, not because it's easy, but because love will give you the strength."* Her words were true. Love for my dad helped me accept the realities of his condition, and with each challenge, I found new ways to adapt. This acceptance became a source of resilience, guiding me through difficult times with compassion and grace.

These stories show that while caregiving can be incredibly challenging, it also reveals strengths we may not have known we possessed.

Lessons Learned from Other Caregivers

Caregivers learn countless lessons along the way, often through trial and error. Learning from others' experiences can provide practical guidance and offer insight into the journey ahead. Here are some of the most valuable lessons I've gathered, both from my own experience and from other caregivers who shared their stories.

1. **Stay Flexible:** One piece of advice I received early on was to "go with the flow." Dementia can be unpredictable, and rigid plans don't always work. For instance, I used to plan every day carefully, but I soon realized my dad's mood could change in an instant. If he wasn't up for his usual routine, I learned to adjust rather than trying to force it. Being flexible made both of our days smoother and allowed me to respond to his needs in the moment.

2. **Learn to Listen Beyond Words:** Another caregiver shared that when her father could no longer speak clearly, she found other ways to *"listen"* to him—through his expressions, gestures, and even his silences. This lesson helped me tremendously as my dad's speech declined. I began paying more attention to his body language and facial expressions, noticing when he was uncomfortable, happy, or simply needed a hand to hold. It taught me that communication is much more than words.

3. **Celebrate Small Joys:** A fellow caregiver once told me, *"Don't wait for big moments to celebrate—find joy in the small things."* One of my favorite memories with my dad happened

during a quiet afternoon when he suddenly started humming an old tune from his youth. I joined in, and we ended up singing together, laughing like we used to. That small moment of joy lifted both our spirits, reminding me that happiness can come even in the most unexpected moments.

4. **Accept Imperfections:** No caregiver is perfect, and mistakes are part of the journey. I remember feeling guilty on days when I didn't have the energy to be as patient as I wanted. Another caregiver shared how she learned to forgive herself for these moments. *"You're doing the best you can,"* she told me, *"and that's enough."* Embracing this helped me let go of unrealistic expectations and focus on the love and effort I put into each day.

These lessons from other caregivers served as a guide for me. They were reminders that caregiving is a learning experience, and each day brings its own wisdom, if we're open to it.

Finding Moments of Happiness in Caregiving

Caregiving for someone with dementia can be challenging, but there are often beautiful, unexpected moments of joy and laughter. These moments not only lift spirits but also create lasting memories that remind us of the love we share.

1. ***A Shared Smile:*** One day, as I was helping my dad get ready for bed, he looked at me, paused, and said with a grin, *"You're pretty good at this, aren't you?"* We both laughed, and I felt this warmth fill my heart. Even in the midst of the daily routine, he recognized my care, and that small acknowledgment was everything. (One thing I usually did was note down these with their dates too. Sometimes when the day was going upside down I just went through my journal and smile) Humor like this, however brief, brought lightness to our day and reminded us of the bond we shared.

2. ***Finding Humor in the Little Things:*** Another caregiver once shared a story about her mother, who had started calling every cat she saw "Fluffy." Whether it was in a book, on TV, or out the window, every cat became "Fluffy." It became an inside joke in their family, and they'd laugh each time she spotted a new "Fluffy." Inspired by her story, I started creating lighthearted moments with my dad by

joking about the small things. Sometimes he'd play along, and these laughs made even the hard days feel a little easier.

3. **Unexpected Surprises**: One of my favorite memories happened on a spring afternoon when my dad, who hadn't danced in years, suddenly grabbed my hand and started moving to an old tune on the radio. His steps were wobbly, but his face lit up with pure joy. We danced for a few minutes, laughing and clapping, and I felt as though time had stopped. These unexpected moments brought us closer and reminded me that even as his memory faded, his spirit remained.

4. **Reconnecting with the Past:** Another caregiver shared how she used to bring out old family photos to spark her husband's memories. Sometimes, he'd remember a detail and surprise her with a story from years ago. Taking her advice, I started doing the same with my dad. One afternoon, while flipping through an album, he recognized a picture of his childhood dog and said, "That's Buster, my best friend." His face softened, and for a moment, it was like the old memories were as fresh as ever. Moments like this brought joy to

both of us, allowing him to reconnect with his past.

These moments of joy and humor were gifts in the caregiving journey. They reminded us that, even amid the challenges, there's still love, laughter, and connection. Caregiving may be demanding, but finding joy in these small moments was what sustained us, day after day.

CHAPTER 12

Resources for Caregivers

Where can caregivers find reliable information and support? Navigating dementia caregiving can feel overwhelming, but thankfully, there are countless resources to help. From insightful books to online support communities and useful apps, these tools can provide essential knowledge, encouragement, and practical assistance. Throughout my journey with my dad, I discovered that having these resources made caregiving a bit less daunting and even brought moments of connection with other caregivers who truly understood the challenges. Here, I'll share some of the most helpful resources that supported our family and made a real difference in our care for him.

List of Trusted Books on Dementia Care

Books on dementia can offer insights, practical tips, and emotional support, helping caregivers understand the experience better. These are some of the most impactful books I found, ones

A Caregiver's Guide for Dementia and Alzheimer's Disease

that offered both practical advice and compassionate guidance.

1. *"The 36-Hour Day" by Nancy L. Mace and Peter V. Rabins*: Often called the "caregiver's bible," this book covers almost every aspect of dementia care, from understanding symptoms to managing behavior changes and navigating healthcare. It provided us with clear explanations and solutions to many challenges we faced, such as how to respond when my dad became disoriented or when he struggled with his memory. This book became our go-to guide, answering questions that seemed to come up daily.

2. *"Learning to Speak Alzheimer's" by Joanne Koenig Coste:* This book helped me rethink how to communicate with my dad as his dementia progressed. Using an approach called "habilitation," it teaches caregivers to adapt to the person's world, focusing on positive reinforcement and flexibility. For instance, instead of correcting him when he became confused, I learned to gently join his reality, making him feel comfortable and understood. The author's perspective shifted how we connected with him, which improved our caregiving relationship.

3. *"Creating Moments of Joy Along the Alzheimer's Journey" by Jolene Brackey:* One of the most inspiring books I read, this guide emphasizes the importance of creating positive, joyful moments, even during difficult times. The author's anecdotes and advice inspired me to find small ways to bring happiness to my dad's day, whether it was by singing his favorite songs or looking through family photos together. This book reminded me that even in advanced stages, there are ways to create connection and comfort.

These books became part of our caregiving "toolkit," providing guidance, encouragement, and a deeper understanding of what my dad was going through. Each page offered a bit of reassurance, making the journey a little lighter.

Websites and Organizations

Websites and organizations dedicated to dementia care provide caregivers with up-to-date information, research, and a community of support. Many of these organizations also offer local services and hotlines, creating a lifeline for families facing the challenges of dementia.

1. **Alzheimer's Association:** The Alzheimer's Association website (alz.org) became one of our most trusted sources for information. It offers articles, webinars, and practical resources on every aspect of dementia care. They also have a 24/7 helpline where caregivers can speak directly with experts for support. We called the helpline during a particularly challenging time and received immediate guidance that made a real difference in managing my dad's care.

2. **Dementia Alliance:** Dementia Alliance is an organization that provides resources and emotional support for dementia caregivers. They offered educational materials and local support programs, which gave us access to information specific to our area. Their online forums also became a place where we could connect with others facing similar challenges, sharing experiences and learning from others' journeys.

3. *Local Alzheimer's and Dementia Groups:* Many communities have local Alzheimer's and dementia support groups, often hosted by hospitals, community centers, or churches. Attending a few meetings in our area allowed us to build connections and gain

support from people who understood the daily ups and downs of caregiving. This local network became an invaluable source of encouragement, especially when we needed to talk to people face-to-face.

4. ***Family Caregiver Alliance***: This nonprofit organization provides a range of caregiver resources, including advice on legal issues, respite care options, and self-care. Their articles helped us navigate complex topics, such as legal planning and finding affordable in-home care. This practical information was crucial in helping us stay organized and prepared for what lay ahead.

These organizations became pillars of support, guiding us with reliable information and connecting us with a wider community. Knowing that help was just a phone call or click away eased some of the stress and uncertainty of caregiving.

Apps and Tools

Smartphone apps are an excellent way to stay organized, track health information, and even find emotional support. These apps became part of our daily routine, helping us manage my dad's care more effectively and freeing up mental energy.

1. **CareZone**: CareZone is an app that allowed us to manage my dad's medications, track symptoms, and store health information all in one place. It also has a reminder function, which ensured we never missed a dose. Whenever we needed to update his doctor, we could pull up his history on the app, which saved us time and helped keep everyone on the same page.

2. **CaringBridge**: CaringBridge is a social network designed specifically for caregivers to update family and friends about a loved one's health journey. We used it to share updates with relatives, posting about my dad's day-to-day progress or memorable moments. It was a convenient way to keep everyone informed without having to make multiple phone calls or send separate messages.

3. **Headspace**: While not specifically for caregivers, the Headspace app offers guided meditations that helped me manage stress. Spending just a few minutes each day using the mindfulness exercises gave me moments of calm amid the chaos of caregiving. This app

became a valuable tool for self-care, reminding me that taking time for myself was essential.

Using these apps helped streamline our daily routines, organize important information, and build a network of support. They provided practical assistance while also creating a sense of connection and calm.

Templates and Checklists

Templates and checklists can simplify caregiving, providing structure to track medications, contacts, and daily routines. These tools were invaluable in our family's journey, as they helped us stay organized and ensured my dad received consistent care. (If you don't have any I have them at the end of the book to make your caregiving journey easy)

1. **Medication Tracker**: Managing my dad's medications was much easier with a printed medication tracker. This template allowed us to record each medication, the dosage, and the schedule. We kept it on the fridge, so everyone in the family knew exactly when and what medications he needed. Having this central list also helped when new caregivers came to assist, ensuring continuity in his care.

2. **Emergency Contacts Sheet**: We created an emergency contacts sheet that listed his doctor's information, the nearest hospital, and family members' phone numbers. This sheet was kept in a visible place so that any family member or caregiver could easily access it. It provided peace of mind, knowing that in an emergency, we could act quickly and efficiently.

3. **Daily Care Routine:** A daily care routine checklist became part of our caregiving routine, breaking down each day into manageable steps. From morning grooming to meal times and evening activities, having a routine checklist helped us keep track of his needs and gave my dad a predictable schedule, which he found comforting.

4. **Symptom Tracker**: A symptom tracker helped us monitor changes in my dad's behavior, sleep, or appetite. This simple template allowed us to note any new symptoms or shifts in mood, which we then shared with his doctor. Tracking symptoms over time helped us identify patterns and adjust his care to make him more comfortable.

Using these templates and checklists brought a sense of organization to our caregiving, making the days run more smoothly and ensuring my dad's needs were consistently met.

These resources provided us with the knowledge, organization, and emotional connection we needed, empowering us to give my dad the best possible care and creating a network of support we could rely on every step of the way.

AT THE END OF THIS GUIDE YOU WILL SEE THESE TEMPLATES SO AS TO MAKE YOUR CAREGIVING JOURNEY EASY.

CHAPTER 13

FAQs and Common Concerns

When caring for someone with dementia, questions constantly come up—about symptoms, safety, communication, and how to handle the emotional toll. I know this from my own experience with my dad, as every day seemed to bring new challenges and uncertainties. This section covers some of the most common questions and concerns, along with practical advice and reassurance drawn from my family's journey.

Answers to Frequently Asked Questions

1. **How do I know if my loved one's forgetfulness is normal aging or dementia?**

<u>Answer</u>: A certain degree of forgetfulness is common with aging—like misplacing keys or occasionally forgetting a name. However, with dementia, the memory loss is more persistent and affects daily life. In my dad's case, we

started noticing he'd forget important things, like whether he had eaten breakfast or where he was going. He'd also repeat the same questions every few minutes. If you're noticing similar patterns or if your loved one is struggling with familiar tasks, it might be time to consult a doctor for a cognitive assessment.

2. How do I properly communicate with an individual who has dementia?

Answer: Communication can be challenging, especially as language and memory fade. The key is to keep it simple and patient. I found that making eye contact, speaking slowly, and using short sentences helped my dad understand and respond better. We avoided arguing or correcting him, and instead tried to validate his feelings. For example, if he was looking for a relative who had passed away, we would gently redirect the conversation instead of correcting him, focusing on keeping him calm and comforted.

3. What are some ways to handle wandering?

Answer: Wandering is a common and potentially dangerous behavior. We started by creating a safer environment at home—using door alarms and ensuring my dad always had an ID bracelet with our contact information. One tip that helped was placing familiar photos around the house, especially near exits, which helped him feel more oriented and reduced his urge to leave. We also tried to keep him engaged with activities he enjoyed, like looking through photo albums or taking short supervised walks, which seemed to satisfy his desire to move around.

4. **Should I try to bring up old memories, or will that confuse my loved one?**

Answer: Bringing up familiar memories can be comforting, especially if they're linked to positive feelings. I found that my dad loved hearing stories from his childhood or looking through old family photos. Sometimes, he'd remember small details, and other times he'd just listen, but it usually put a smile on his face. However, if certain memories bring frustration or confusion, it's best to focus on the present and find simple activities that bring comfort.

A Caregiver's Guide for Dementia and Alzheimer's Disease

5. ***How do I handle difficult behaviors, like aggression or anger?***

Answer: Behavioral changes are common in dementia, and they're often tied to feelings of frustration, confusion, or fear. If my dad became angry or upset, I learned that staying calm was essential. Speaking softly and giving him space to cool down usually helped. Over time, we also identified some triggers, like loud noises or feeling rushed, which allowed us to prevent many outbursts by keeping his environment calm and predictable.

These FAQs address just a few of the challenges that come up in dementia caregiving. The answers are rooted in both personal experience and advice from other caregivers, offering a practical approach to everyday questions.

Handling Caregiver Concerns

1. ***How can I keep my loved one safe without making them feel confined?***

Answer: Safety was a big concern for us, especially as my dad became less aware of his surroundings. We focused on creating a safe environment by adding nightlights, removing tripping hazards, and securing doors. We wanted him to feel free within his space, so instead of restricting him, we set up areas where he could move around safely. For instance, we designated certain rooms for his walks and activities, and he seemed to enjoy the sense of independence without the risks of wandering outside.

2. *How do I take care of my own health while caregiving?*

Answer: Caring for someone with dementia is demanding, and it's easy to neglect your own needs. I learned the hard way that self-care is non-negotiable. Taking breaks, whether through respite care or asking family members to step in, made all the difference. Even small things, like having a quiet cup of tea or taking a short walk, helped me recharge. Over time, I realized that maintaining my health wasn't just good for me, it made me a more patient and effective caregiver for my dad.

3. *How do I handle family disagreements about my loved one's care?*

Answer: Caregiving can strain family dynamics, especially when everyone has their own opinions. We experienced this when my siblings and I disagreed on certain care decisions. We found that open communication was crucial. Having regular family meetings helped us stay aligned on my dad's needs and allowed everyone to voice concerns. We also reminded ourselves that, while we might disagree, we all wanted what was best for him. When tensions rose, focusing on his well-being helped us set aside differences and work as a team.

4. *How do I manage guilt about needing breaks or feeling frustrated?*

Answer: Feeling guilty is a common issue for caregivers, especially when you need time for yourself or feel exhausted. I went through periods where I felt guilty if I didn't have the energy to be as patient as I wanted. However, I learned that these feelings are natural and that being a caregiver doesn't mean being perfect. Accepting help, taking breaks, and forgiving yourself for moments of frustration are essential. Each of these actions, I realized, actually made me a better caregiver, as they allowed me to approach my dad with a refreshed mindset.

5. *How do I deal with the grief of losing my loved one gradually?*

<u>Answer</u>: The grief that comes with dementia caregiving is unique because it's a slow loss that happens over time. Watching my dad change was heartbreaking, and I had to come to terms with "losing" parts of him while he was still alive. I found comfort in remembering the good times and focusing on the things that still connected us, like sharing old stories or listening to his favorite songs together. Talking to others in support groups who were going through similar experiences also helped me process this gradual grief and reminded me that I wasn't alone.

These FAQs and common concerns reflect the complexities of dementia caregiving. The journey comes with countless questions, many without simple answers. (Yes, because I'm still hurting from losing my dad) But by sharing these insights and learning from others, caregivers can find practical solutions, emotional support, and a sense of community. In the end, caregiving is about love, resilience, and finding ways to make each day a little brighter—for the person you're caring for and for yourself.

Conclusion

The journey of caregiving for a loved one with dementia is like no other—a path that tests, teaches, and transforms. As I reflect on my time caring for my dad, I realize just how much this experience has changed me. It was a journey full of challenges, requiring patience and compassion that often seemed impossible to sustain. Yet, in the end, it was also a journey full of meaning, connection, and love. Caregiving taught me that resilience isn't about never feeling tired or discouraged; it's about showing up, day after day, with love, even when things are difficult. This chapter is a tribute to you, the caregiver, who has given so much of yourself in this journey.

Caregivers are often the unsung heroes, quietly carrying the weight of responsibility and love. Every caregiver's journey is unique, shaped by their loved one's needs and by the caregiver's own strength and dedication. Looking back, I see so many moments with my dad that tested my limits but also taught me patience in ways I never imagined. It wasn't only about tending to his needs; it was also about finding ways to bring comfort, joy, and respect to his life.

I remember one night in particular when I felt exhausted, with seemingly no energy left to give. My dad, sensing my weariness, reached out and patted my hand, as if to say, *"You're doing just fine."* That small gesture reminded me of the impact of caregiving—the bond that deepens even in moments of exhaustion. Those little reminders of why we care can carry us through the hardest days. If you're reading this and have cared for a loved one, know that your role is invaluable and deeply honored. The love you give changes lives, including your own, in profound and lasting ways.

If I could share one piece of advice with you, it would be to find moments of kindness toward yourself as well as toward the person you're caring for. This journey is filled with ups and downs, and self-compassion will be your greatest ally. There will be days when you feel completely drained, and that's okay. Those are the times to remind yourself that you are only human and that you're doing the best you can.

As you move forward, embrace the small victories and moments of peace, even if they're fleeting. The simple joys—the warmth of a shared laugh, the comfort of a gentle touch—these are the moments that make caregiving meaningful. There is no "perfect" way to care for someone with dementia; there's only the love and patience you bring to each day. Carry that with you as a reminder that every effort, every small act of care, truly matters.

And remember, you're not alone on this journey. Reach out to others, lean on family and friends, and don't hesitate to seek support when you need it. Just as you are there for your loved one, there are others ready to be there for you.

When the caregiving journey comes to an end, it brings a mix of emotions—grief, relief, and sometimes a loss of identity. I went through this myself after my dad passed away. I felt both the heaviness of loss and a strange emptiness, not knowing what to do with the time that was once dedicated to his care. It was a new chapter that required me to turn some of that caregiving energy back onto myself.

The transition can be challenging, but remember that self-compassion is key. Allow yourself time to grieve, rest, and reconnect with parts of yourself that may have been put on hold. Find activities that bring you peace and fulfillment, whether it's reading, gardening, (I'm back to my garden now. I abandoned it to care for my dad) spending time with loved ones, or enjoying simple stories that make you smile. I found comfort in reading familiar children's Bible stories, as they brought me a sense of calm and inspiration. Sometimes, revisiting these gentle stories can offer caregivers and patients alike a way to unwind and reconnect with simple, comforting messages of faith and love.

This new chapter is also an opportunity to reflect on all you have learned. Caregiving changes us, often bringing out strengths we didn't know we had. Embrace these lessons, and know that they will carry you forward. Whether you choose to continue helping others or explore new paths, this journey has given you the strength that will serve you well in whatever comes next.

In closing, I hope this book has offered you the knowledge, support, and encouragement to face the many challenges of caregiving with a bit more confidence and compassion. If these pages have helped you feel seen, understood, or better equipped, I'd be honored if you'd share your thoughts in a review. Your feedback not only supports other caregivers but also builds a community of understanding and encouragement.

Thank you for joining me on this journey, for your dedication, and for the compassion you bring to caregiving. May you find peace, joy, and strength in your path forward, and may you always remember the profound impact you have made in your loved one's life.

GLOSSARY

1. **Dementia**: A general term for symptoms affecting memory, thinking, and social abilities that interfere with daily life. It is not a specific disease but rather a group of conditions, including Alzheimer's disease.

2. **Alzheimer's** Disease: The most common form of dementia, characterized by memory loss, confusion, and personality changes due to the degeneration of brain cells.

3. **Cognitive Decline:** A gradual decrease in cognitive abilities, such as memory, problem-solving, and language skills, often seen in dementia.

4. **Sundowning**: Increased confusion, agitation, or restlessness that occurs in people with dementia, typically in the late afternoon or evening.

5. **Power of Attorney (POA):** A legal document that grants someone authority to make decisions on behalf of another person, especially when they can no longer make decisions independently.

6. **Palliative Care:** Medical care focused on relieving symptoms, pain, and stress, improving the quality of life for people with serious illnesses, including dementia.

7. **Plaques**: Abnormal clusters of protein fragments (beta-amyloid) in the brain associated with Alzheimer's disease.

8. **Tangles**: Twisted fibers of a protein called tau that build up inside brain cells in Alzheimer's disease.

9. **Neurological**: Related to the brain, spinal cord, and nerves.

10. **Neurodegenerative**: Describes conditions where nerve cells in the brain or nervous system gradually lose function.

11. **Memory Loss:** The inability to recall information or past events.

12. **Aphasia**: Difficulty with language, including speaking, reading, or understanding speech.

13. **Apraxia**: Loss of ability to perform familiar movements or tasks despite physical ability.

14. **Agnosia**: Inability to recognize objects, people, sounds, or smells.

15. **Wandering**: The tendency of individuals with dementia to walk away or become lost.

16. **Caregiver Burnout**: Physical, emotional, and mental exhaustion from caregiving responsibilities.

17. **Neuropathology**: Study of diseases of the nervous system.

18. **Aggression**: Hostile or violent behavior, common in advanced stages of dementia.

19. **Agitation**: Restlessness or irritability often triggered by confusion or discomfort.

20. **Paranoia**: Irrational fear or mistrust of others.

21. **Hallucinations**: Seeing or hearing things that aren't there.

22. **Delusions**: False beliefs held despite evidence to the contrary.

23. **Anxiety**: Excessive worry or fear, often triggered by unfamiliar situations.

24. **Depression**: Persistent feelings of sadness or loss of interest, common in early stages.

25. **Emotional Lability:** Rapid and unpredictable changes in emotions.

26. **Person-Centered Care:** An approach focusing on the individual's preferences, values, and needs.

27. **Activities of Daily Living (ADLs):** Basic self-care tasks like eating, bathing, and dressing.

28. **Advanced Directive:** Legal document specifying a person's wishes for medical care.

29. **Respite Care**: Temporary relief for primary caregivers through professional or volunteer services.

30. **Validation Therapy:** A communication approach acknowledging and respecting the person's feelings and reality.

31. **Reminiscence Therapy**: Therapy encouraging recall of past events to stimulate memories and emotional connection.

32. **Behavioral Interventions**: Strategies to address challenging behaviors.

33. **Care Plan:** A detailed approach to caring for someone with dementia.

34. **Cognitive Stimulation Therapy (CST):** Activities designed to improve mental functioning.

35. **Memory Aids:** Tools like labeled pictures, notes, or calendars to assist with memory.

36. **Assistive Technology:** Devices like GPS trackers or alarms to ensure safety and independence.

37. **Life Story Work**: Using personal photos, documents, and stories to maintain a sense of identity.

38. **Neurotransmitters**: Chemicals in the brain that transmit signals, affected in dementia.

39. **Hydration**: The process of maintaining adequate fluid levels, crucial for those with dementia.

40. **Nutritional Support:** Tailored diet plans to maintain physical health.

FREE GIFT

Thank you for reading this book and I believe that you learnt a lot. **Congratulations** on getting to this page now **HERE** is your **REWARD**.

A Caregiver's Guide for Dementia and Alzheimer's Disease

Emergency Contact Sheet

EMERGENCY CONTACT LIST

DATE: * ★ * _____

Instructions: Fill in the necessary information below.

Under Contact Type, identity of the person is a PRIMARY DOCTOR or a FAMILY MEMBER.

S/N	Name	Contact Type	Phone Number	Address

A Caregiver's Guide for Dementia and Alzheimer's Disease

EMERGENCY CONTACT LIST

DATE: * ★ * ―――――――

Instructions: Fill in the necessary information below.

Under Contact Type, identity of the person is a PRIMARY DOCTOR or a FAMILY MEMBER.

S/N	Name	Contact Type	Phone Number	Address

A Caregiver's Guide for Dementia and Alzheimer's Disease

Medication and Healthcare Tracking Templates

Healthcare Tracker

Date: _____ Doctor: _____

Information Report

Purpose

Observations

Next Step

Daily Health Check

Sleep: _____ hrs (☐ Good ☐ Fair ☐ Poor)

Meals: ☐ Breakfast ☐ Lunch ☐ Dinner ☐ Snacks

Appetite: ☐ Good ☐ Average ☐ Poor

Hydration: _____ mL

Bowel/Bladder: ☐ Normal ☐ Irregular Notes: _____

Physical Activity: ☐ None ☐ Light ☐ Moderate ☐ Intense

A Caregiver's Guide for Dementia and Alzheimer's Disease

Healthcare Tracker

Date: _____ Doctor _____

Information Report

Purpose

Observations

Next Step

Sleep: _____ hrs (☐ Good ☐ Fair ☐ Poor)

Meals: ☐ Breakfast ☐ Lunch ☐ Dinner ☐ Snacks

Appetite: ☐ Good ☐ Average ☐ Poor

Hydration: _____ mL

Bowel/Bladder: ☐ Normal ☐ Irregular Notes: _____

Physical Activity: ☐ None ☐ Light ☐ Moderate ☐ Intense

DAILY HEALTH CHECK

A Caregiver's Guide for Dementia and Alzheimer's Disease

Symptoms Tracker

Symptoms and Behaviour Tracker

Date: _____   Week: _____

Symptoms and Behaviours	Sun	Mon	Tue	Wed	Thu	Fri	Sat
1 _____	○	○	○	○	○	○	○
2 _____	○	○	○	○	○	○	○
3 _____	○	○	○	○	○	○	○
4 _____	○	○	○	○	○	○	○
5 _____	○	○	○	○	○	○	○
6 _____	○	○	○	○	○	○	○
7 _____	○	○	○	○	○	○	○
8 _____	○	○	○	○	○	○	○
9 _____	○	○	○	○	○	○	○
10 _____	○	○	○	○	○	○	○
11 _____	○	○	○	○	○	○	○
12 _____	○	○	○	○	○	○	○
13 _____	○	○	○	○	○	○	○
14 _____	○	○	○	○	○	○	○
15 _____	○	○	○	○	○	○	○

Cognitive: ☐ Confused ☐ Forgetful ☐ Oriented

Mood: ☐ Calm ☐ Anxious ☐ Agitated

Behavior: ☐ Normal ☐ Wandering ☐ Aggressive

Physical: ☐ Pain ☐ Fatigue ☐ Other: _____

A Caregiver's Guide for Dementia and Alzheimer's Disease

Symptoms and Behaviour Tracker

Date: _____   Week: _____

Symptoms and Behaviours	Sun	Mon	Tue	Wed	Thu	Fri	Sat
1 _____	○	○	○	○	○	○	○
2 _____	○	○	○	○	○	○	○
3 _____	○	○	○	○	○	○	○
4 _____	○	○	○	○	○	○	○
5 _____	○	○	○	○	○	○	○
6 _____	○	○	○	○	○	○	○
7 _____	○	○	○	○	○	○	○
8 _____	○	○	○	○	○	○	○
9 _____	○	○	○	○	○	○	○
10 _____	○	○	○	○	○	○	○
11 _____	○	○	○	○	○	○	○
12 _____	○	○	○	○	○	○	○
13 _____	○	○	○	○	○	○	○
14 _____	○	○	○	○	○	○	○
15 _____	○	○	○	○	○	○	○

Cognitive: ☐ Confused ☐ Forgetful ☐ Oriented

Mood: ☐ Calm ☐ Anxious ☐ Agitated

Behavior: ☐ Normal ☐ Wandering ☐ Aggressive

Physical: ☐ Pain ☐ Fatigue ☐ Other: _____

A Caregiver's Guide for Dementia and Alzheimer's Disease

Medication Tracker

MEDICATION TRACKER

Month: _____

Dosage	Name of Medicine	Time	Notes

A Caregiver's Guide for Dementia and Alzheimer's Disease

MEDICATION TRACKER

Month: _____

Dosage	Name of Medicine	Time	Notes

A Caregiver's Guide for Dementia and Alzheimer's Disease

Caregiver's Checklist

Caregiver's Checklist

Self Regulation Ideas for _____

Before I explode, I will

Date: _____

Circle some ideas you will try.

Get a drink	Draw a picture	Take calming breaths
Take a walk	Talk with someone	Take a break

What helped you calm down today? _____
_____
_____
_____

A Caregiver's Guide for Dementia and Alzheimer's Disease

Caregiver's Checklist

Self Regulation Ideas for _____

Before I explode, I will

Date: _____

Circle some ideas you will try.

Get a drink	Draw a picture	Take calming breaths
Take a walk	Talk with someone	Take a break

What helped you calm down today? _____
_____
_____
_____
_____

A Caregiver's Guide for Dementia and Alzheimer's Disease

CONVERSATIONAL QUESTIONS

1. What has been the most rewarding part of your caregiving journey so far, and how has it shaped your relationship with your loved one?

_____

_____

_____

_____

_____

2. What strategies have you found most helpful for managing stress and maintaining your well-being as a caregiver?

_____

_____

_____

_____

_____

3. How do you approach communicating with your loved one when they are confused or unable to express themselves clearly?

_____

_____

_____

4. What resources or tools have made the biggest difference in your ability to provide effective care?

_____

_____

A Caregiver's Guide for Dementia and Alzheimer's Disease

5. **Can you share a moment where you felt overwhelmed and how you managed to navigate through it?**

6. **How do you balance caregiving responsibilities with your personal life, and what boundaries have you set to avoid burnout?**

7. **What advice would you give to someone who is just beginning their caregiving journey for a loved one with dementia or Alzheimer's?**

A Caregiver's Guide for Dementia and Alzheimer's Disease

_____

_____

8. Have you noticed any creative or unexpected ways that your loved one communicates emotions or memories? How do you respond?

_____

_____

_____

_____

_____

9. What coping mechanisms or routines have you developed to deal with the emotional challenges of caregiving?

_____

_____

10. **If you could change one thing about the support system for caregivers, whether it's from healthcare providers, family, or society, what would it be?**

About The Author

Jenny Daniels is an author inspired by her father's journey through dementia and Alzheimer's. Driven by love and a desire to help others, she writes compassionate guides offering practical advice and emotional support to caregivers. Jenny's work highlights the challenges of caregiving while celebrating the meaningful connections and moments of joy it brings.

THANK YOU!

Thank you for purchasing and reading this book. I'm happy to share my experience with you, but I need a favour from you.

If this book touched your life, I'd love to hear your honest review, it helps others find it too

Share it with friends, family, or anyone who might benefit. And don't miss my other books designed to inspire and uplift your journey.

Your support means everything. Thank you!

INDEX

A
Aggression 93, 165

B
Bathing and grooming assistance 25, 35, 52, 53, 75, 82,

Behavioral changes. 93

Books and educational materials. 106, 153

C
Caregiver checklist. 16, 159, 160, 189, 190

Caregiver resources. 69, 74, 75, 76, 157

Communication strategies. 54, 71, 72, 91, 92, 100

D
Dementia-friendly environments. 57

Diagnosis. 58, 58, 60

Dressing Challenges 34, 40, 53, 54, 76, 83, 84

E
Early detection methods. 48, 55, 56

Emergency planning 160, 181

Emotional support 69, 74, 130, 131, 137

End-of-life care. 56, 113, 133

G
Grief 14, 24, 25, 33, 139, 140, 141, 143

Guardianship 119, 120, 121

H
Hospice care. 135, 136

I
Incontinence. 88, 89

L
Legal and Financial Planning. 24, 66, 112, 114, 122

Lewy body dementia. 41, 43

Local support networks 67, 74, 156,

Long-term care insurance

M
Managing wandering 13, 91, 93, 94, 163, 166

Medical appointments 11

Memory Loss. 38, 39, 41, 43, 48

Mild cognitive impairment (MCI). 50, 51, 52

O
Online forums for caregivers. 74, 75, 131

P
Power of attorney.
56, 66, 113

R
Respite care. 70, 115, 129, 134

S
Self-care for caregivers 128

Symptoms of Alzheimer. 40

T
Tracking. 62, 65, 160

W
Will and trust. 113

www.ingramcontent.com/pod-product-compliance
Lightning Source LLC
Chambersburg PA
CBHW071533220526
45469CB00003B/766